Cooking for Family & Friends

★

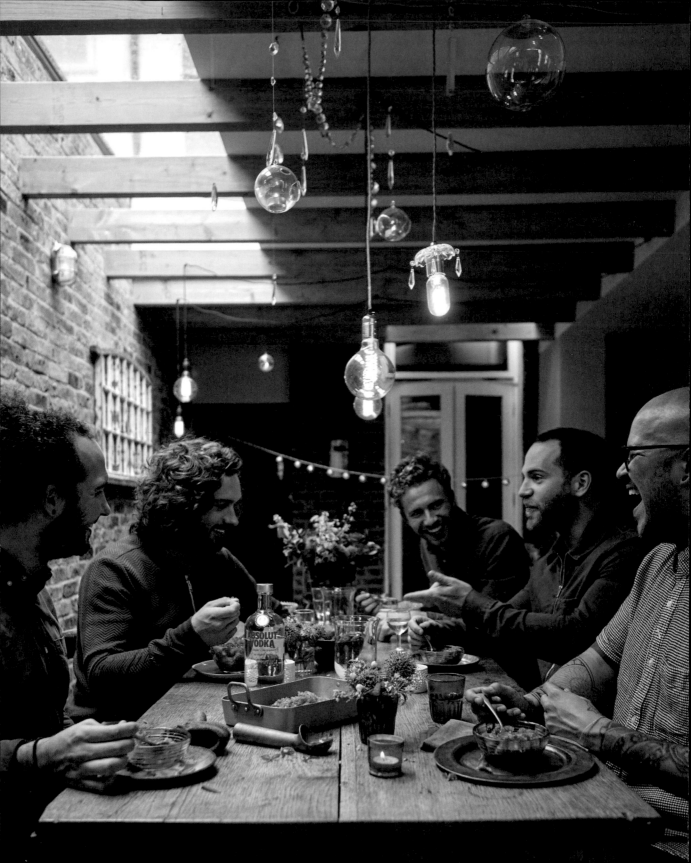

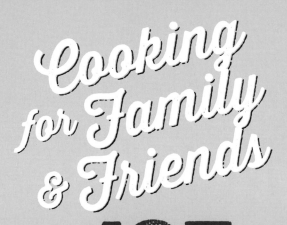

Cooking for Family & Friends

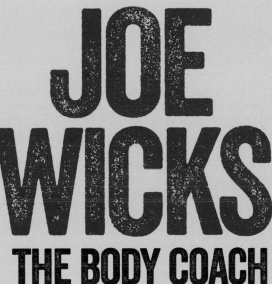

JOE WICKS

THE BODY COACH

100 lean recipes to enjoy together

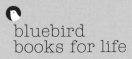

bluebird
books for life

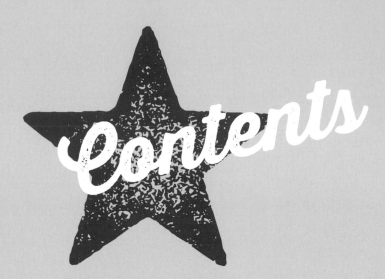

Contents

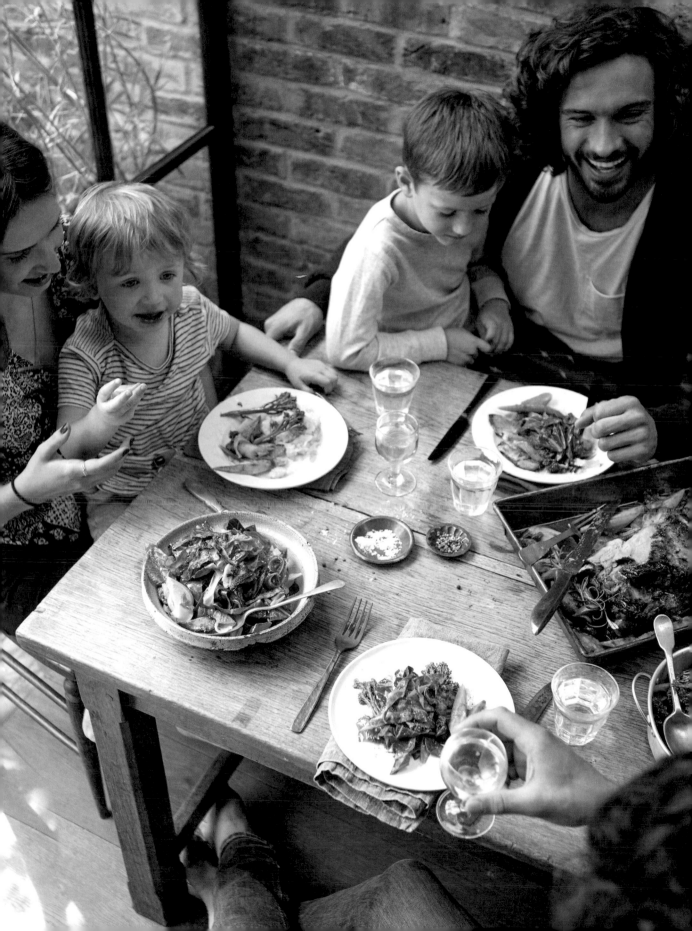

Hello WELCOME TO *COOKING* FOR FAMILY & FRIENDS

First, I would like to say thank you for choosing my new book. I'm really excited to be sharing these new recipes with you. Since day one, it's been my aim to get more people cooking healthy food at home, and I believe this book will do just that. The recipes are tasty and easy to make, and as I've designed them to serve 4–6 people, you and the whole family can enjoy them and stay lean together!

I haven't included any workouts in the book, so this one is all about the food. There are some proper banging recipes in here, such as toad in the hole and beef stew with dumplings – home-cooked classics that remind me of my Nanny Kath. I used to stay with her after school sometimes and she used to fatten me right up until I fell asleep on the carpet in front of the fire. I love how food can bring you such good memories.

You'll notice that some of the recipes, such as my pulled pork and Sunday roasts, take longer to make than my signature 15-minute meals, but I promise they're worth the wait. I've done my best to keep the prep times low, so once that's done you can bung them in the oven, put your feet up and relax or fit in a sneaky workout.

I've also thrown in a couple of my favourite naughty treats too. These pub classics, such as sticky toffee pudding and chocolate fondant, are so not lean. LOL! Oh well, guilty as charged. I don't recommend eating them every day, but we all deserve a treat now and again.

➡ LET'S GET EVERYBODY LEAN

I think there is a big misconception that when you are trying to get lean and eat healthier, it isolates you from your friends and family. I think that could be the case for people following a really low-calorie restrictive diet but I'm not about that life. That's not

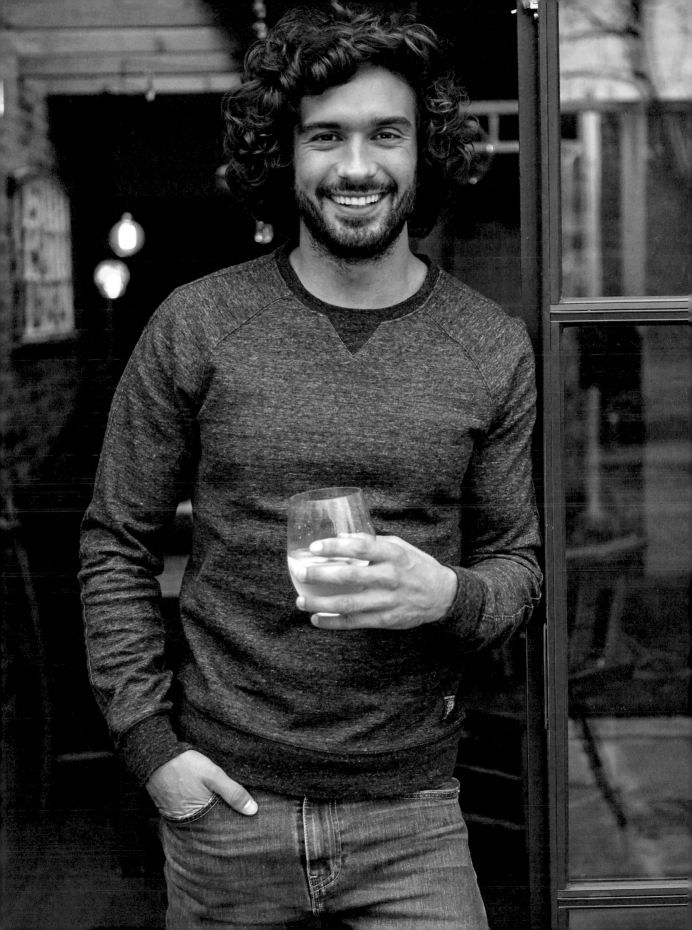

enjoyable or sustainable. I don't believe in low-calorie diets and I don't believe you need to spend your day eating boring meals out of lunch boxes, cooking separate meals for yourself or avoiding meals out with friends and family altogether.

With these recipes, I'm going to show you that eating healthy can be fun and inclusive for everyone at every occasion – even parties, barbecues and Sunday lunches.

➡ START 'EM YOUNG

I believe that kids should be involved in the food choices at home and educated as early as possible about good nutrition and exercise. It's a really important time for them, and it will help shape their health and their future.

When I was growing up, my mum didn't have a clue about nutrition and healthy cooking, and my cupboards were always full of junk food. We rarely sat together as a family and ate. I pretty much lived off sandwiches, pasta with tomato sauce, sweets and cereal. This seemed normal to me at the time but now I know there is a much healthier way to live. I think it's never too early to get kids started in the kitchen.

To get the kids involved, you could get them to help you write shopping lists and fill the baskets at the supermarket. These may seem like small things but I think they could have a big impact.

➡ CAN I GET LEAN WITHOUT EXERCISING?

Although I haven't included workouts in this book, I wanted to talk briefly about the importance of exercise when trying to maintain a healthy body. If you're someone who struggles to stay active and can't bear the thought of going to the gym, then this message is for you.

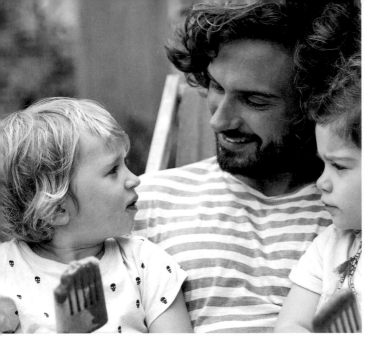
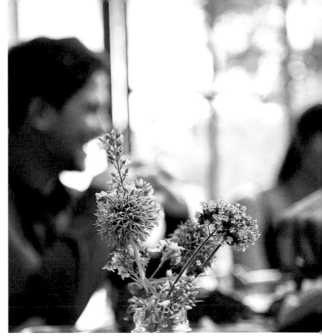
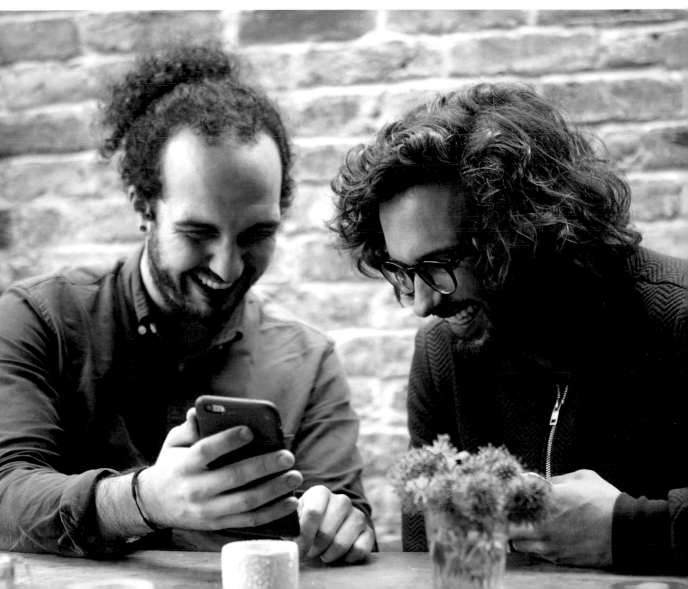

I'm a big believer in doing home workouts and I also believe it's never too late to get lean. You don't need a gym or lots of expensive equipment to get fit. I have a YouTube channel called The Body Coach TV where I share free workouts, which you can do anywhere, at any time. To build strong lean muscle and have a fit healthy heart, you need to work for it, because it just won't come by itself. Plus, if you workout, you can enjoy more of the foods you love!

Many of the meals in here are high in calories, and the reason I don't list them is because I don't think people should obsessively count calories. That said, in order to burn body fat you do need to be burning more calories than you are consuming, so if you want to actually see changes in your body, get moving and try to make exercise a part of your life. There's no need to try to get by on a really low-calorie diet when,

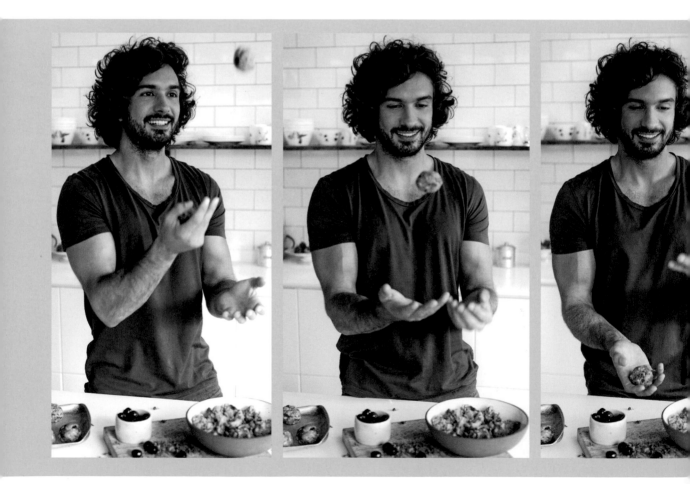

instead, you can exercise, feel good and eat the meals from this book knowing you are making progress.

Exercise isn't just going to make you feel and look better. It's also going to give you more energy and confidence. My advice is to aim for 25 minutes of exercise, four to five days per week.

➡ WHAT SHOULD I BE EATING & WHEN?

The recipes in this book are broken down into five chapters: Reduced Carb, Post Workout, On the Side, Starters & Snacks and Smoothies & Sweet Treats.

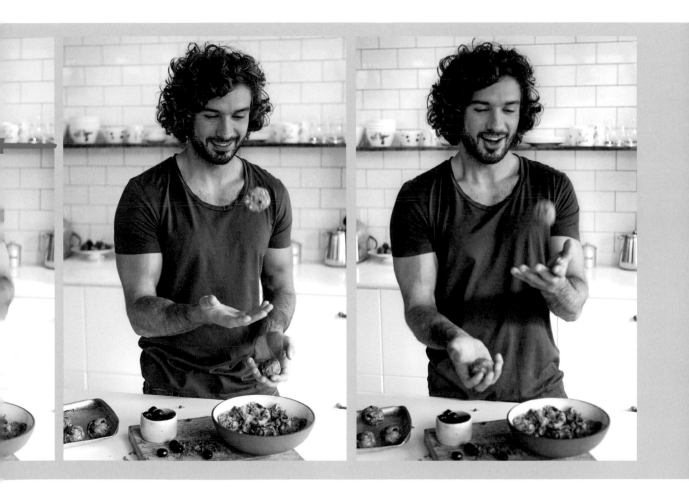

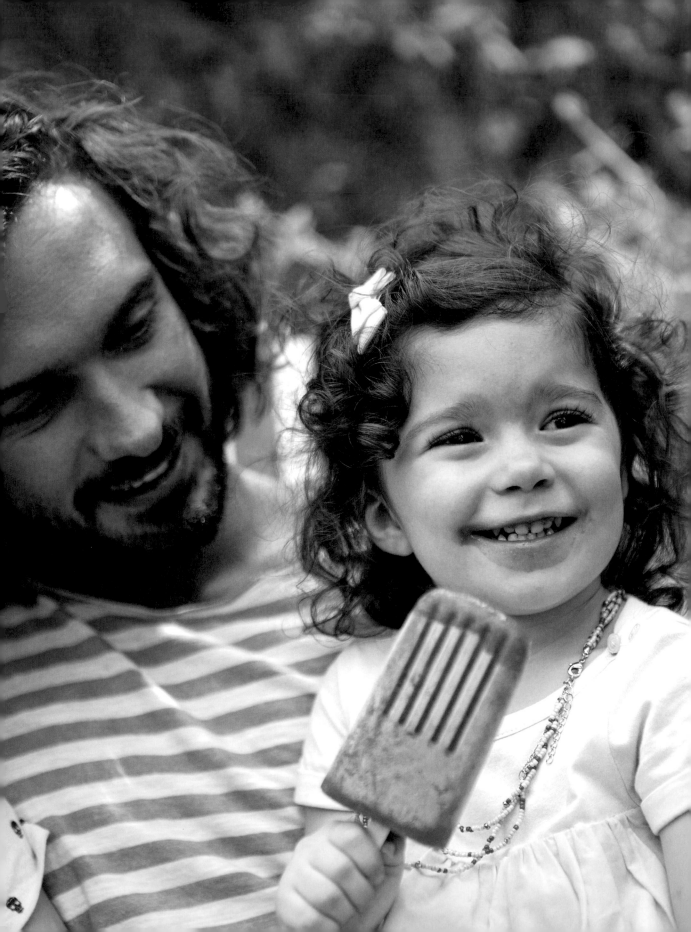

Reduced-carbohydrate meals are higher in healthy fats and proteins. These types of meals are brilliant to have on rest or less active days.

The post-workout meals contain protein and carbohydrates but are lower in fat. These meals are ideally consumed after exercise or on more active days.

I personally consume three reduced-carb meals on a rest day and two reduced-carb meals and one post-workout meal on a training day. I find this a really simple and effective way of staying lean, as I am fuelling my body with the right energy source at the right time.

One thing to be aware of is your portion sizes. Everyone is different and will have different energy demands. For example, if you are an active twenty-year-old exercising five days per week, you will need more food than someone who is forty and doesn't exercise much. The key here is to eat to feel energized – so simply increase or decrease your portions accordingly. Once you get that bit right, you'll find it very easy to sustain a healthy lifestyle and a lean body, all year round.

Good luck! I hope you enjoy the recipes in this book. I'm really proud of it and love seeing my little nephew Oscar making his debut appearance at just seven days old. I believe this book can help your whole family get leaner and healthier. Hopefully you'll be inspired to try out some of my workouts, too.

Lots of love,
Joe ★

STAY IN TOUCH

🐦 📘 👻 📷 @thebodycoach
▶️ The Body Coach TV
thebodycoach.com

Reduced Carb

The recipes in this section are lower in carbohydrates and higher in healthy fats and protein. They will provide your body with a steady source of energy and keep your blood-sugar levels stable. This means you won't be crashing or craving sugars or caffeine to get you through the day.

On a rest day I suggest eating three of these recipes, and on a training day I suggest eating two recipes from this chapter, and one from the Post Workout chapter (see pages 106–181) after you train. Eating this way will make you feel awesome and provide your body with the essential fats to keep you fit and healthy. Don't miss out on my Chicken, chorizo and cauliflower tray bake (see page 32). ★

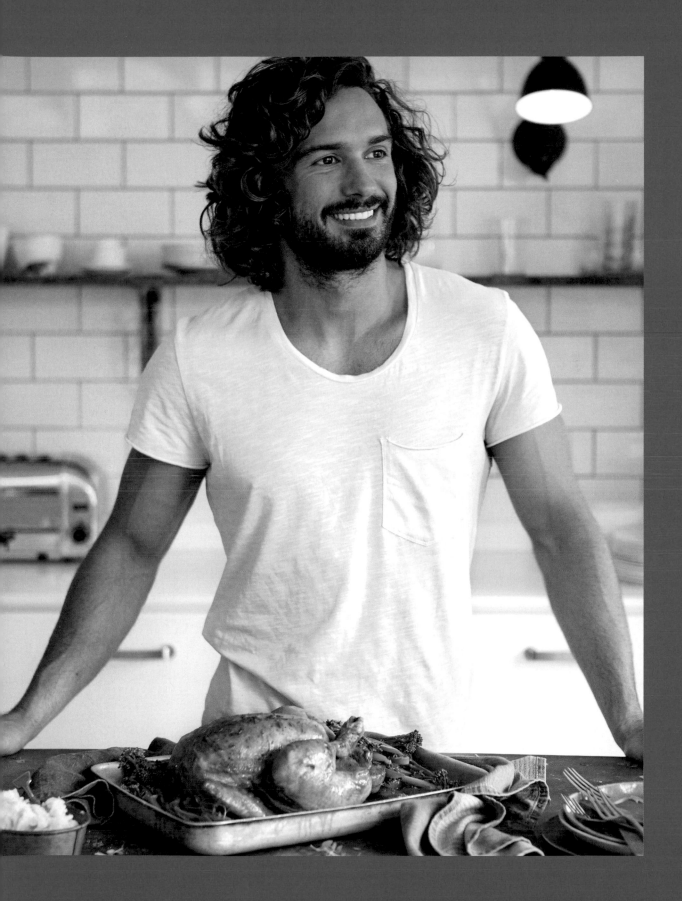

REDUCED-CARB

MY SPANISH SAUSSIE

If you like a bit of Spanish sausage this one is perfect for you. It's basically a one-tray breakfast that everyone can dig into. The chorizo gives this dish all its flavour but if you prefer normal sausages, feel free to swap them.

◆**PREP 10 MINS**
◆**COOK 30 MINS**

4 chorizo sausages, cut into 2cm chunks

2 tbsp coconut oil

300g kale, stalks removed

500g chestnut mushrooms, brushed clean and roughly chopped into quarters

8 eggs

5 spring onions, finely sliced

65ml double cream

25g parmesan, grated

small bunch of chives, finely sliced

Equipment
23 x 18cm baking dish

Preheat your oven to 190°C (fan 170°C/gas mark 5).

Place the sausages into a dry frying pan over a medium to high heat. As the sausages begin to fry, the fat will run out of them. Cook the sausages for about 5 minutes, or until they are golden brown and almost cooked through.

Melt 1½ tablespoons of the coconut oil in a second saucepan over a medium to high heat. When it is hot, add the kale and mushrooms and cook, stirring regularly for about 7 minutes, or until the kale has wilted and the mushrooms are almost cooked through.

Use the remaining coconut oil to grease the baking dish and then place the chorizo sausages, kale and mushrooms in the dish, mixing it all up. Make eight small indents in the mixture and crack the eggs directly into the holes. Sprinkle the spring onions over the top.

Pour the cream over the mixture, sprinkle over the parmesan and slide the dish into the oven to bake for 15 minutes.

Remove the bubbling dish from the oven, sprinkle with chopped chives and serve straight out of the baking dish.

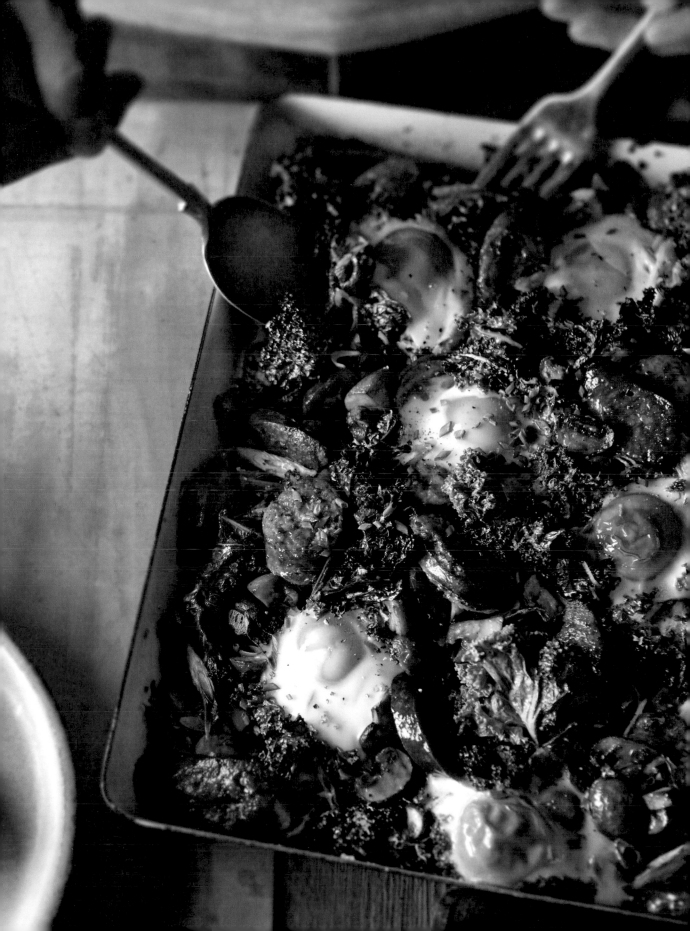

REDUCED-CARB

EASY EGGS & HAM

This is one of my favourite quick and easy breakfasts for any day of the week. It is way more nutritious than a bowl of cereal or slice of toast: proper fuel to set you up for the day. Just be sure to get some good-quality ham and not the cheap reformed stuff.

◆PREP 10 MINS
◆COOK 10 MINS

large knob of butter
1 large leek, finely chopped
1 red chilli, finely sliced, plus a little extra to garnish
200g good-quality thick-cut ham, roughly chopped into 2–3cm chunks
150g frozen peas
75ml chicken stock
large handful of baby spinach
4 eggs
4–5 tbsp grated mature cheddar

Melt the butter in a large frying pan over a medium to high heat. When it is bubbling, slide in the leek and chilli and fry, stirring occasionally for 3 minutes, or until the leek just starts to soften.

Crank up the heat to maximum and add the ham and frozen peas. Stir-fry for 1 minute and then pour in the stock and bring to the boil.

Simmer until the peas are fully heated through, then drop in the spinach and stir it in. Reduce the heat to medium and create four rough indents in the mixture. Carefully crack an egg into each hole and sprinkle the grated cheese over the top.

Slide a lid (or a large plate if you don't have a lid) over the mixture and leave to cook like this for 3 minutes for a soft yolk.

You can either share this straight from the pan, or carefully divide it between two plates. Scatter with a little more chilli and get stuck in.

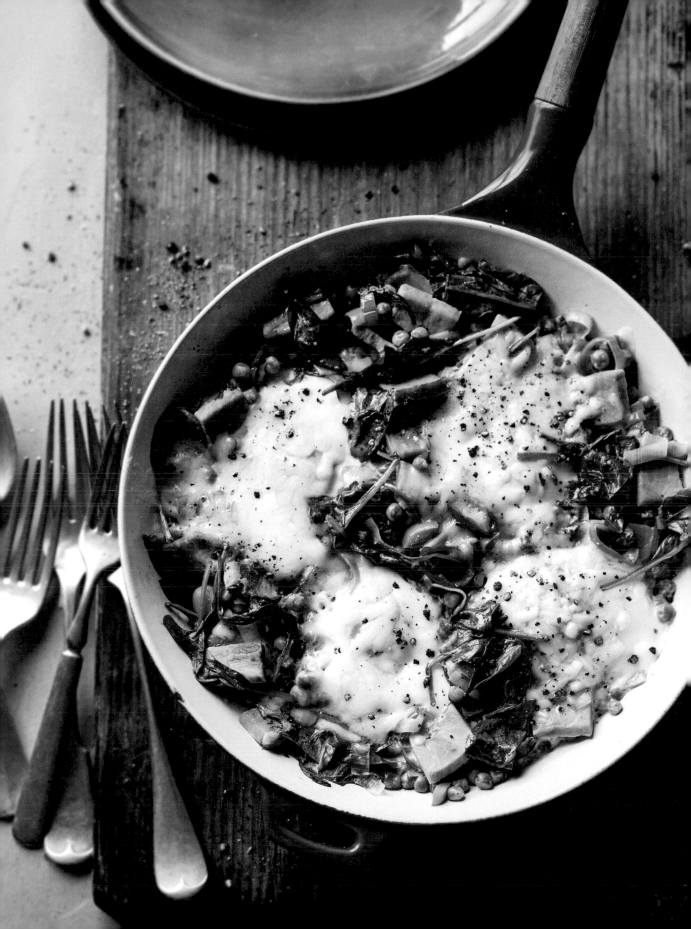

Serves 2

REDUCED-CARB

BAKED EGGS & SALMON

This is a real lean-muscle-building breakfast. It's quick, easy and full of healthy fats. The crème fraiche and spinach are perfect alongside the smoked salmon. Enjoy!

⬥PREP 5 MINS
⬥COOK 10 MINS

1 knob of butter
2 spring onions, finely sliced
90g smoked salmon, roughly cut into 1cm slices
2 large handfuls of baby spinach
2 tbsp crème fraiche
black pepper
2 eggs
3 tbsp grated cheddar
1 red chilli, de-seeded and finely sliced
2 tbsp breadcrumbs

Preheat your oven to 180°C (fan 160°C/gas mark 4).

Melt ½ knob of butter in an ovenproof frying pan over a medium to high heat. When it is bubbling, chuck in the spring onions and fry for 1 minute. Add the sliced smoked salmon and the spinach and cook until the spinach has fully wilted down.

Reduce the heat to medium and splodge in the crème fraiche along with a good grinding of black pepper. Stir the crème fraiche into the pan until it has melted to make a creamy sauce.

Make two rough indents in the mixture and crack an egg into each one. Sprinkle the cheese over the eggs and then slide the pan into the oven to cook for 5 minutes.

While the eggs are in the oven, melt the remaining butter in a frying pan over a high heat. Add the sliced red chilli and breadcrumbs to the pan and fry them until the breadcrumbs are golden and crisp.

Remove the pan from the oven, sprinkle the fried chilli and breadcrumbs over the top and serve.

★ *IF YOU DON'T HAVE AN OVENPROOF FRYING PAN, USE A NORMAL FRYING PAN. WHEN YOU'VE STIRRED IN THE CREME FRAICHE, TRANSFER THE WHOLE THING TO AN OVENPROOF DISH, CRACK IN THE EGGS AND BAKE FOR 12–15 MINUTES.*

Serves 4

REDUCED-CARB
→BBQ

GRILLED PRAWN & HALLOUMI SALAD

OMG, I love a bit of grilled squeaky cheese. It may seem odd grilling the watermelon but it tastes wicked with the salty halloumi. If you're not a fan of prawns you could always use grilled chicken instead.

→PREP 10 MINS
→COOK 10 MINS

600g raw prawns, peeled and cleaned

flesh of ½ small watermelon (about 600g), cut into triangles

250g halloumi, cut into 12 slices

bunch of basil, leaves only, roughly torn

bunch of mint, leaves only, roughly torn

3 tbsp toasted pine nuts

14 pitted black olives

4 large handfuls of rocket

1 lemon, cut into wedges

drizzle of olive oil, to serve

Fire up the barbecue, if using.

Cook the prawns, watermelon and halloumi separately on the hot barbecue or using a hot griddle pan. Each ingredient will take roughly 2 minutes to cook on each side on the barbecue. If you're using a griddle pan, the prawns will need longer: around 2½ minutes on each side. Cook the prawns first, making sure they are totally pink all the way through, then the watermelon, and finally the halloumi, so it remains warm when you serve the salad.

When you have cooked the prawns, watermelon and halloumi, toss them together in a bowl with the basil, mint, pine nuts, olives and rocket.

Serve the salad with the lemon wedges and a glug of olive oil.

SEE PHOTOS OVERLEAF ➡

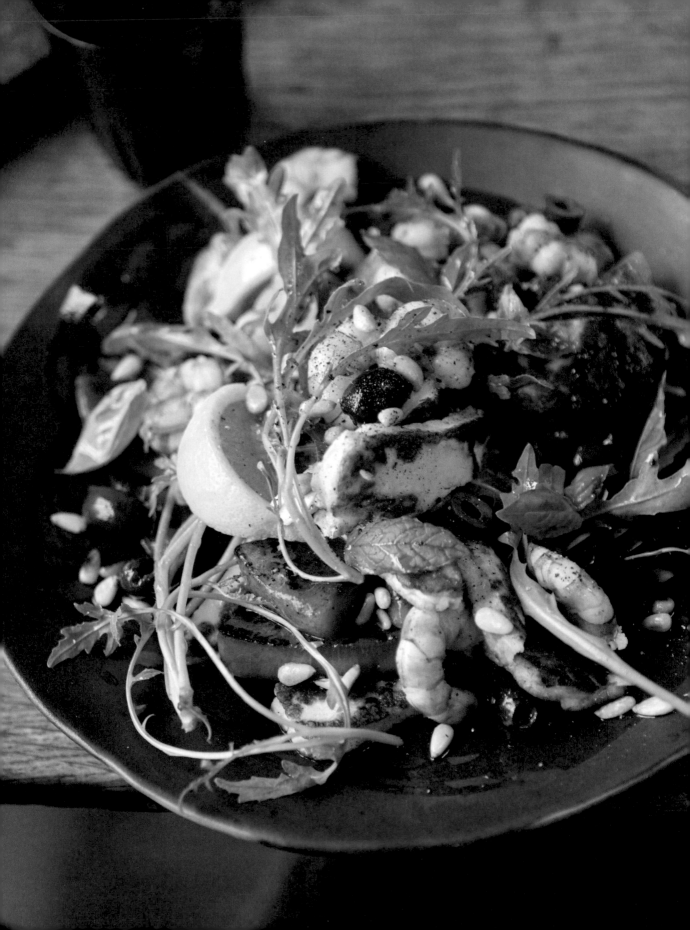

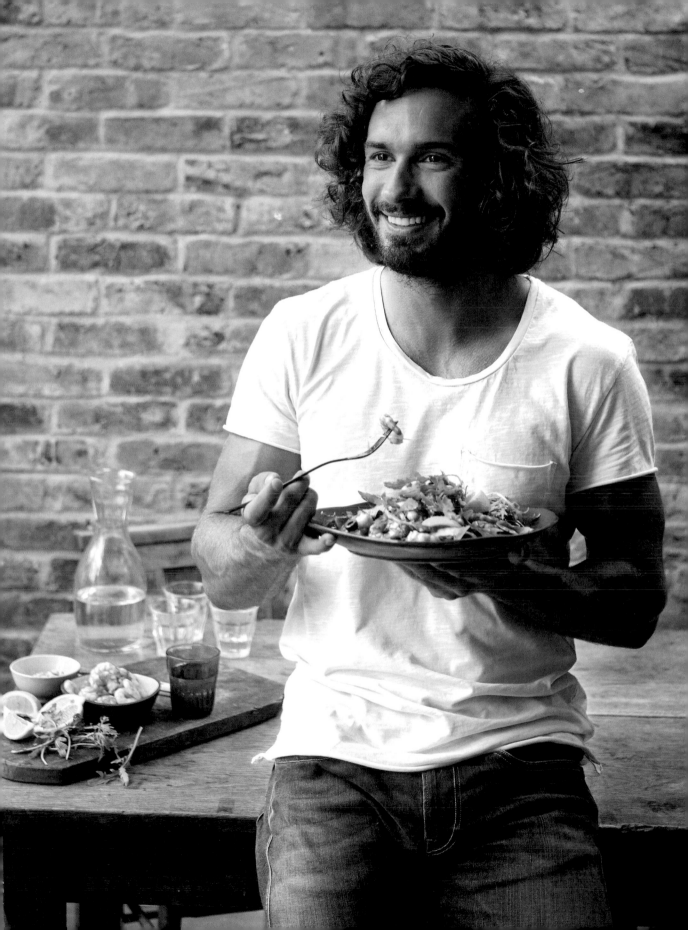

REDUCED-CARB

PARMA HAM, FIG & GOAT'S CHEESE SALAD

If you're a cheese lover, you'll know that figs and parma ham are a perfect match. And you can't really go wrong with a bit of creamy goat's cheese.

◆PREP 10 MINS
◆COOK 25 MINS

2 red onions, cut into 1cm wedges

1 tbsp balsamic vinegar, plus a little extra to drizzle

1 tbsp olive oil

4 x 100g soft goat's cheese rounds

6 figs, cut into quarters lengthways

4 large handfuls of rocket

60g walnuts, roughly chopped

8 slices of parma ham

Preheat your oven to 200°C (fan 180°C/gas mark 6).

Scatter the red onion wedges in a baking tray and drizzle with the balsamic vinegar and olive oil. Toss them in the oil and vinegar, slide the tray into the oven and roast for 20 minutes, turning once halfway through.

Remove the tray from the oven and lay the four cheese rounds on top. Scatter over the fig quarters and then slide the tray back into the oven. Roast for a further 5 minutes, until the cheese has softened.

Divide the rocket over four plates and top with the baked goat's cheese, red onions and roasted figs. Finish by scattering the walnuts over the top and piling the parma ham on the side. Drizzle with a little more balsamic vinegar and dig in.

REDUCED-CARB

SALMON, PRAWN & AVOCADO SALAD

This is a great recipe full of healthy fats to give you lots of energy. It looks awesome on one big serving plate that everyone can get stuck into.

➡PREP 15 MINS
➡COOK 20 MINS

300g salmon fillet, skin-on

6 tbsp olive oil

2 gherkins, drained and finely chopped

2 large shallots, finely diced

1½ tbsp capers, roughly chopped

3 lemons

salt and pepper

1 iceberg lettuce, shredded

2 avocados, de-stoned and cut into wedges

1 x 110g ball of mozzarella, drained

12 cherry tomatoes, roughly halved

16 cooked king prawns

30g shelled pistachios, roughly chopped

small bunch of dill, finely sliced

small bunch of chives, finely sliced

Bring a pan of water to the boil over a high heat.

When the water is boiling, slide in the salmon fillet, place a lid on top and reduce the temperature to its lowest setting. Leave the fish to cook like this for 15 minutes, then take the pan off the heat and leave it in the water for 5 minutes.

Carefully remove the fillet from the pan, peel off the skin and then leave to cool completely.

To make the dressing, mix together the olive oil, chopped gherkins, shallots, capers and the juice of one lemon. Season with a little salt and pepper.

Spread the shredded lettuce over a large plate and place the avocado wedges over the top. Break up the cooked salmon into large chunks with a fork and dot around the plate. Tear the mozzarella into chunks and scatter on top along with the cherry tomatoes and king prawns.

Squeeze over the juice of another lemon and then spoon or drizzle the dressing all over the salad. Cut the remaining lemon into wedges. Sprinkle over the chopped pistachios, dill and chives and serve with the lemon wedges.

Serves 4

REDUCED-CARB
→MAKE AHEAD

CHICKEN & MOZZARELLA SALAD WITH WARM TOMATO DRESSING

This is probably the best salad I've ever made. Poaching the chicken in stock keeps it really moist and gives it so much more flavour. I think your family and friends will love this one.

→PREP 15 MINS
→COOK 20 MINS

1.25 litres chicken stock

4 skinless chicken breasts

5 tbsp olive oil

3 spring onions, finely sliced

2 large sprigs of rosemary, needles only

1 large clove garlic, finely chopped

1 red chilli, de-seeded and finely sliced

16 cherry tomatoes, roughly halved

salt and pepper

6 tbsp breadcrumbs

2 avocados, de-stoned and cut into wedges

2 x 110g balls of mozzarella, torn into large chunks

To serve

2 large handfuls of rocket

1–2 tbsp balsamic vinegar

Pour the chicken stock into a large lidded saucepan and bring it to the boil. Slide in the chicken breasts – if the liquid doesn't cover them then add a little more stock or water. Bring back up to the boil, clamp on the lid and then reduce to a low heat.

Cook the chicken breasts on a very low simmer for 10 minutes, then remove the pan from the heat and leave the chicken in the warm stock for a further 10 minutes with the lid still on.

Meanwhile, make the dressing. Pour 4½ tablespoons of the oil into a saucepan and add the spring onions, rosemary, garlic, red chilli and tomatoes along with a good grinding of salt and pepper. Place the saucepan over a medium to low heat and cook for 10 minutes, being sure not to let the oil get too hot. Turn off the heat and leave the mixture to sit while you prepare the rest of the salad.

Heat the remaining ½ tablespoon of oil in a large frying pan over a medium to high heat. When it is hot, tip in the breadcrumbs and fry for about 3 minutes, or until they are crisp and golden. Transfer the breadcrumbs to a clean piece of kitchen roll to drain off the excess oil.

Carefully remove the cooked chicken from the stock and tear it up with your hands or a couple of forks. Place the chicken onto a large serving plate along with the avocado and mozzarella chunks. Spoon over the warm tomato dressing, then top with the rocket and the fried breadcrumbs. I like to serve this salad with a little balsamic vinegar on the side.

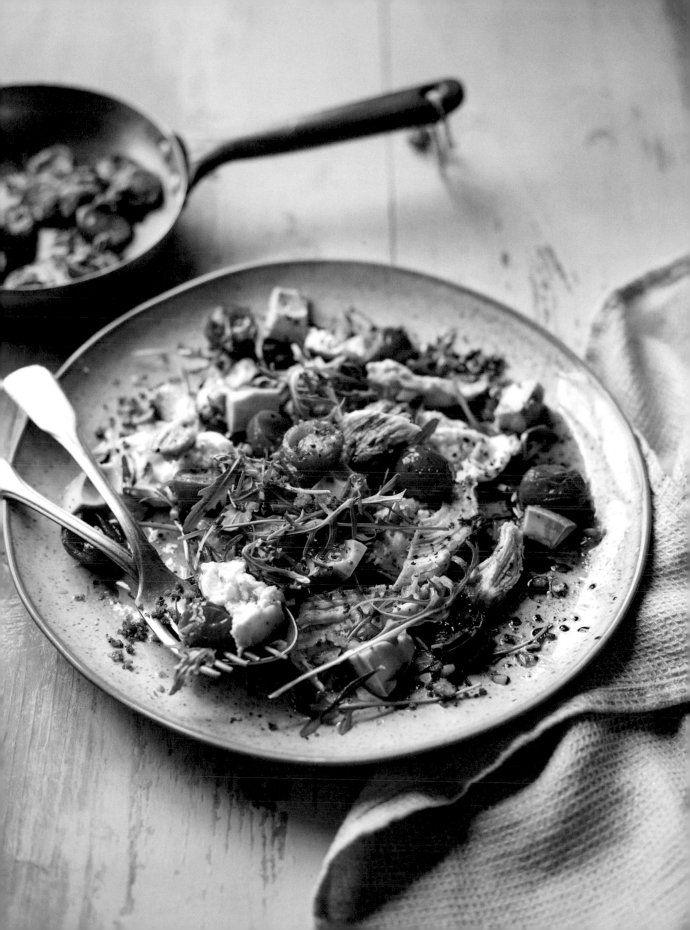

REDUCED-CARB

TERRY THE TUNA WITH QUICK PICKLED RADISHES & CUCUMBER

This looks fancy but it is really easy to make and tastes amazing. Be sure to prep like a boss by getting your cucumbers and radishes pickled in advance. They will keep for up to 3 days covered in the fridge.

**➔PREP 15 MINS,
   PLUS PICKLING TIME
➔COOK 15 MINS**

2 cucumbers, peeled
200g radishes, cut into 3mm slices
2 large shallots, cut into thin rings
salt
65ml rice wine vinegar
½ tbsp coconut oil
4 x 190g tuna steaks
4 large handfuls of rocket
100g feta
small bunch of dill
1½ tsp nigella seeds – optional

Turn the cucumbers into long, thin ribbons by peeling off whole lengths of each one from top to bottom, putting a little more pressure on the peeler than you normally would.

Keep peeling on one side until you reach the watery seeds, then turn the cucumber 90-degrees and begin peeling again. Repeat the process until all you are left with is a watery core. Place the ribbons into a bowl.

Add the radishes and shallots to the bowl with a pinch of salt. Pour in the vinegar and toss the whole lot together using your hands or a couple of wooden spoons. Cover the salad with cling film and leave in the fridge to pickle for an hour.

About 10 minutes before the pickling time is up, melt the oil in a large frying pan over a high heat. If you only have a small frying pan then use half the oil and cook the tuna in two batches. Don't overcrowd the pan.

When the oil is very hot, season the tuna steaks with salt and carefully lay them into the pan. Fry them for 90 seconds on each side and then slide them out and blot them with kitchen roll to remove any excess oil. Leave the fish to rest until you're ready to eat.

Drain and lightly squeeze the pickled veg to remove as much liquid as possible. Add the rocket to the bowl and toss the whole lot together. Divide the salad over four plates, then crumble over the feta. Sit the cooked tuna steaks alongside and top with a few sprigs of dill and the nigella seeds, if you fancy it.

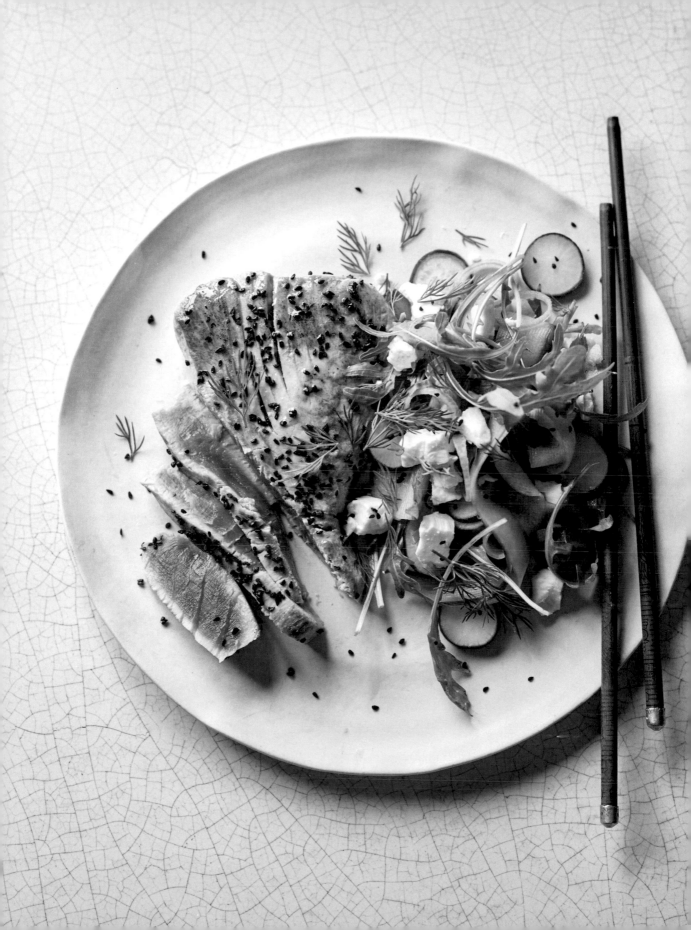

Serves 2

REDUCED-CARB

BURRATA WITH MINT PESTO

If you love mozzarella but haven't tried burrata you really should give it a try. It's probably the best cheese in the world and takes creaminess to a whole new level.

▶PREP 10 MINS

large bunch of basil, leaves only
large bunch of mint, leaves only
½ bunch of chives, roughly chopped
17g pine nuts
4 tbsp olive oil
1½ tbsp sherry vinegar
15g parmesan, grated
2 balls of burrata

To serve
rocket
2 slices of parma ham

Equipment
food processor

To make the pesto, place the basil, mint, chives, pine nuts, olive oil, sherry vinegar and parmesan into a small food processor and blitz until smooth.

Take two plates and place a ball of burrata onto each one, then scatter it with a few rocket leaves. Lay down a slice of ham on each serving and top with the pesto. Bosh!

★ *YOU CAN SAVE LEFTOVER MINT PESTO AND ADD IT TO A GRILLED CHICKEN SALAD, OR STIR IT THROUGH PASTA FOR AN EASY POST-WORKOUT MEAL.*

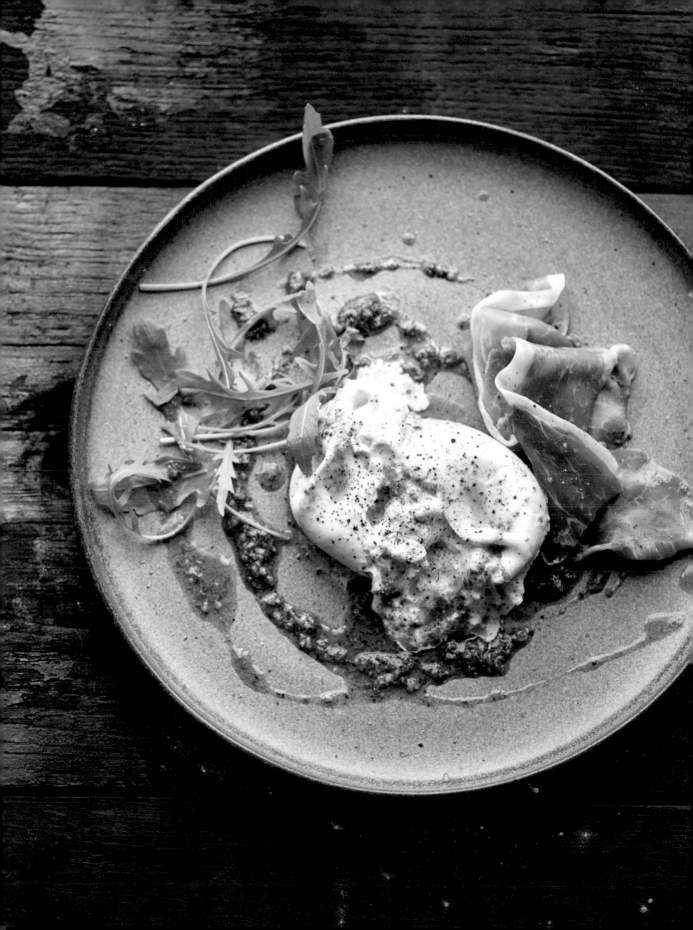

REDUCED-CARB

CHICKEN, CHORIZO & CAULIFLOWER TRAY BAKE

This is one of those meals that is well worth the wait. It tastes incredible and everything gets thrown in the same tray. I recommend preheating the oil in the roasting tray to get the chicken skin nice and crispy.

➡**PREP 12 MINS**
➡**COOK 40 MINS**

2 tbsp olive oil

4 chicken breasts, skin-on

1 cauliflower, florets only (roughly 500g)

1 red onion, cut into 12 wedges

150g cooking chorizo, cut into 1cm pieces

4 sprigs of thyme

16 cherry tomatoes, preferably on the vine

2 large handfuls of baby spinach

Preheat your oven to 190°C (fan 170°C/gas mark 5).

When the oven is hot, pour the oil into a roasting tray and slide it into the oven. Leave the tray to heat up for 10 minutes.

When the oil is nice and hot, carefully slide the tray out of the oven and lay the chicken breasts in it, skin-side down. Tumble the cauliflower florets around the breasts and put the tray back into the oven to roast for 10 minutes.

Remove the tray from the oven and scatter over the red onion, chorizo and sprigs of thyme. Return the tray to the oven and roast for a further 15 minutes.

Take the tray out again, flip over the chicken breasts and give all the vegetables a bit of a stir.

Place the tomatoes on top of the mixture and give the whole lot one more 10-minute blast in the oven.

Remove the tray from the oven and while it is hot, drop the spinach on top and carefully stir it through so it wilts a little in the heat. Serve.

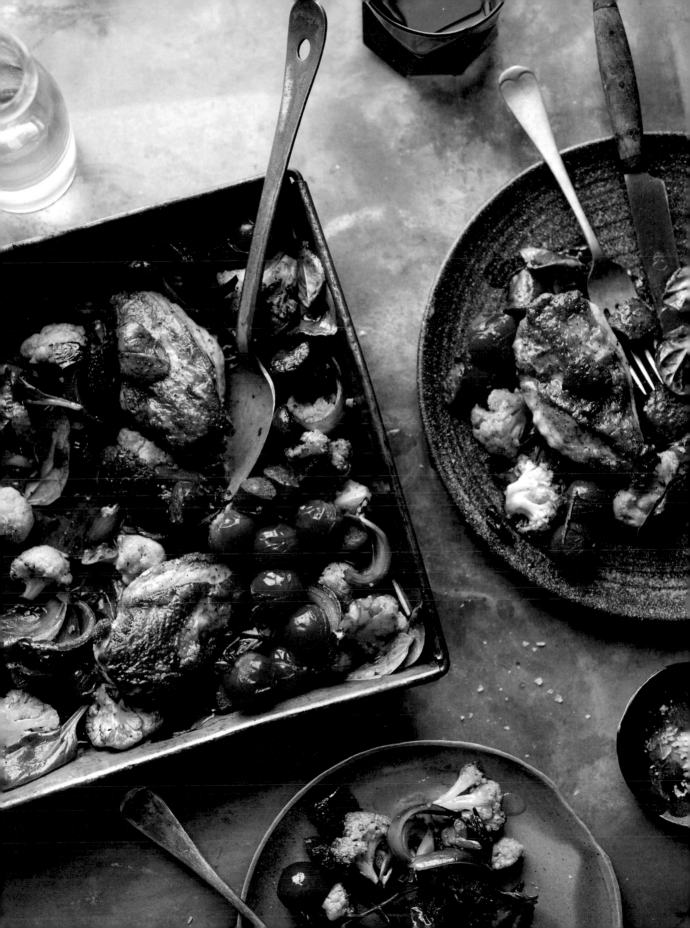

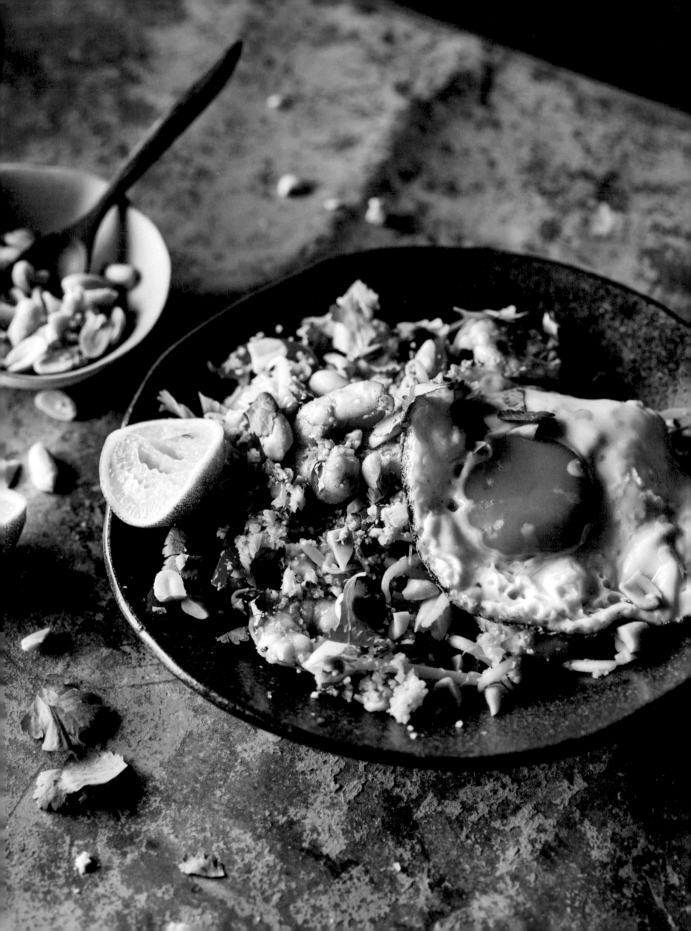

REDUCED-CARB

PRAWN & CAULIFLOWER RICE STIR-FRY

I wasn't too sure about cauliflower rice to begin with but I'm a massive fan now. You basically blitz it up until it looks like rice and it makes a great low-carb alternative for your meals.

→PREP 15 MINS
→COOK 10 MINS

1 small cauliflower, florets only (about 400g)

1 tbsp coconut oil

4 spring onions, finely sliced

2 cloves garlic, finely chopped

1 courgette, grated

1 red pepper, cut into 5mm slices

400g raw prawns, peeled and cleaned

2 chillies, de-seeded and finely sliced

150g beansprouts

2 tsp light soy sauce

½ tbsp kecap manis sauce

To serve
small bunch of coriander, roughly chopped

75g peanuts, roughly chopped

4 fried eggs

juice of 1 lime, plus extra wedges

Equipment
food processor

Place the cauliflower florets into a food processor and blitz them until they are roughly the size of rice grains. Set aside.

Melt the coconut oil in a large frying pan or wok over a high heat. Add the spring onions, garlic, courgette and red pepper and stir-fry for about 2 minutes, or until the vegetables start to soften.

Chuck in the prawns and continue to stir-fry for 2 minutes, or until the prawns start to turn from grey to pink – it is not necessary for the prawns to be totally cooked through at this point. Scrape in the cauliflower rice and continue to stir-fry the whole lot together for 3 minutes.

By now the prawns should be cooked through and the vegetables should have softened but still have a bit of texture. Turn off the heat and toss through the chillies, beansprouts, soy sauce and kecap manis sauce.

Divide the stir-fry between four plates or bowls and serve it topped with the coriander, peanuts, a fried egg each and a good squeeze of lime juice.

REDUCED-CARB
→GOOD TO FREEZE

CHICKEN & AUBERGINE BALTI

If like me you love a curry night, then this one will be right up your street. Cooking the chicken thighs on the bone does take a bit longer, but it adds so much more flavour to the final dish.

→PREP 15 MINS
→COOK 40 MINS

2 tbsp coconut oil

2 red onions, diced

½ tsp fenugreek seeds

3 green cardamom pods, bashed

2 red peppers, cut into 2–3cm chunks

2 medium aubergines, cut into 2–3cm chunks

10 skinless chicken thighs, bone-in

4 tsp garam masala

1 tsp ground coriander

1 tsp ground turmeric

1 tsp paprika

1 tbsp tomato puree

300ml chicken stock

225g paneer, cut into 2cm cubes

1 red chilli, de-seeded and finely sliced

salt and pepper

juice of ½ lemon

large bunch of coriander, roughly chopped

Melt 1½ tablespoons of the coconut oil in a large hob-proof casserole dish or saucepan over a medium to high heat. When it is hot, add the red onions and cook for 3 minutes. Add the fenugreek and cardamom and continue to cook for 2 minutes.

Add the red peppers, aubergines and chicken thighs to the dish or saucepan and fry the whole lot together for 3–4 minutes, or until the chicken is more white than pink. Sprinkle in 3 teaspoons of the garam masala and all of the ground coriander, turmeric and paprika. Fry the mixture, stirring almost constantly for 1 minute, then squeeze in the tomato puree, continuing to stir-fry for another minute.

Pour in the stock and bring to the boil, put a lid on top and cook the curry for 30 minutes or until the chicken is cooked through. Check by cutting into one of the thickest pieces to make sure the meat is cooked all the way through, with no raw pink bits left.

About 10 minutes from the end of cooking, melt the remaining ½ tablespoon of coconut oil in a frying pan over a medium to high heat. When it is hot, add the paneer cubes and fry them for about 2 minutes, turning regularly until they are lightly browned. Reduce the heat and add the red chilli and the final teaspoon of garam masala.

Give the paneer one final toss, season it with salt and pepper, and pour in the lemon juice. Tip the paneer into the curry and cook for 5 minutes. Just before serving, stir through the chopped coriander.

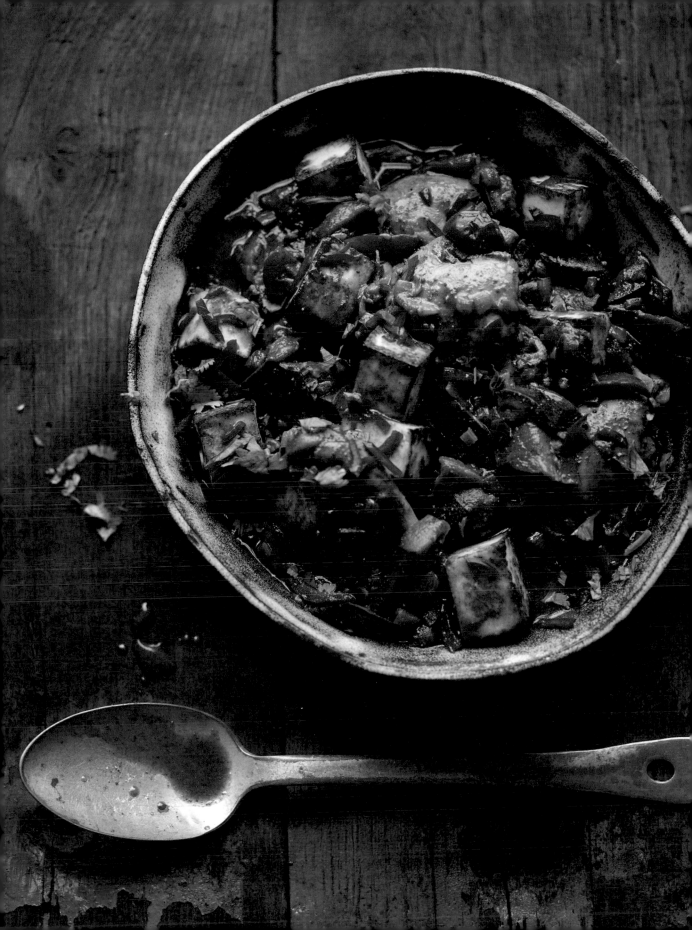

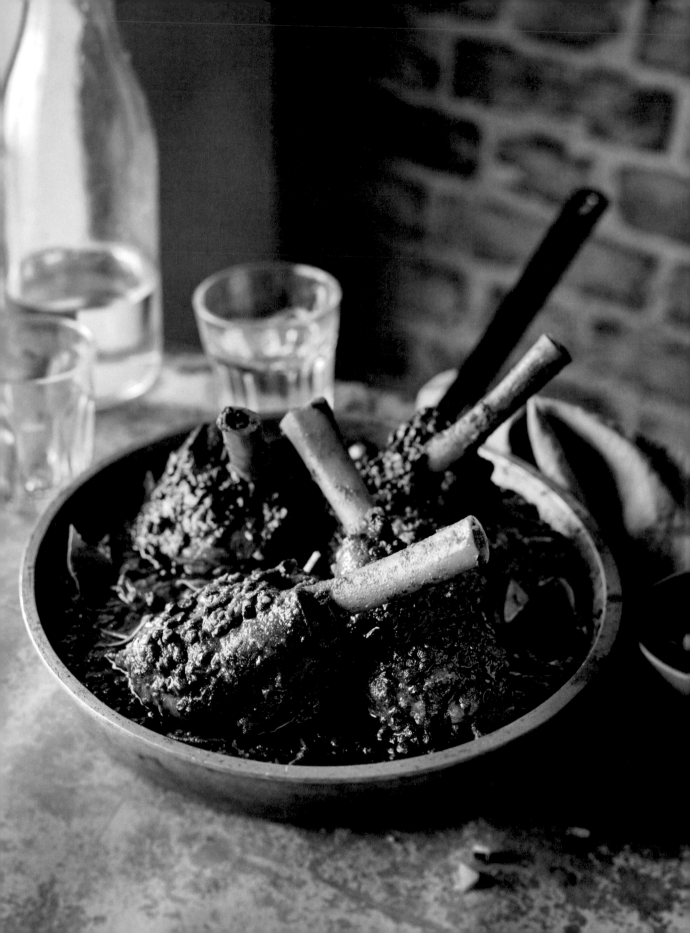

REDUCED-CARB
➡LOW & SLOW
➡GOOD TO FREEZE

THE LAMB-SHANK REDEMPTION

This saag is a real melt-in-the-mouth dish when cooked low and slow. An added bonus is that the shank is one of the cheapest cuts of lamb. Don't be fooled by its price though, as it tastes incredible.

➡**PREP 10 MINS**
➡**COOK 2 HRS 10 MINS**

2 red onions, roughly diced
2 tbsp coconut oil
5 cloves garlic, finely chopped
5cm fresh ginger, finely chopped
1 tbsp garam masala
½ tbsp ground turmeric
½ tbsp ground coriander
¼–½ tbsp chilli powder – depending on if you like it hot
2 tbsp tomato puree
1 bay leaf
750ml chicken stock
4 lamb shanks
150g ready-to-eat puy lentils
200g baby spinach
large bunch of fresh coriander, roughly chopped
tomato, red onion and cucumber salad, to serve

Equipment
food processor

Chuck the diced onions into a food processor and blend until almost completely smooth.

Melt the oil in a large saucepan over a medium to high heat. When it is hot, scrape in the blitzed onion. Cook the onion, stirring regularly for about 8 minutes, until softened and lightly coloured. Add the garlic and ginger and continue to stir-fry for a further 2 minutes. If the mixture starts to burn or stick to the bottom of the pan, pour in a splash of water and reduce the heat a little.

Sprinkle in the garam masala, turmeric, ground coriander and chilli powder, and cook, stirring almost constantly for 30 seconds. Squeeze in the tomato puree, drop in the bay leaf and then continue stirring and cooking for a further minute.

Pour in the chicken stock and bring to the boil. Carefully lay the lamb shanks into the mixture.

Clamp a lid tightly on the pan and leave to cook for 45 minutes over a low heat. Then remove the lid, flip the shanks over and give the sauce a stir to make sure it isn't sticking to the bottom of the pan. Replace the lid and keep on cooking for a further hour, giving it a little stir every now and then.

When the shanks have cooked for 1 hour 45 minutes, they should be very tender. Slide in the lentils and cook for a further 15 minutes without the lid, by which time the lentils should be very soft.

Drop in the baby spinach and let it wilt in the heat. Take the pan off the heat and stir through the fresh coriander. Serve the saag with a chunky tomato, red onion and cucumber salad.

REDUCED-CARB
➤**LOW & SLOW**
➤**GOOD TO FREEZE**

LAMB MADRAS CURRY

There's nothing better than a night in with good friends and a home-cooked curry. This one is really easy to make and lamb makes a nice change from the usual chicken.

➤**PREP 15 MINS**
➤**COOK 1 HR 45 MINS**

1½ tbsp coconut oil
2 onions, finely diced
3 tsp jarred garlic puree
3 tsp jarred ginger puree
120g madras spice paste
1.25kg lamb neck, trimmed of fat and then cut into 3cm chunks
250ml chicken stock – optional
100g cashew nuts
1 small cauliflower, florets only (about 500g; large florets cut in half)
125g ready-to-eat puy lentils
260g baby spinach
large bunch of coriander, roughly chopped

Equipment
blender

Melt the coconut oil in a large saucepan or casserole dish over a medium to high heat. When it is hot, slide in the diced onions and fry, stirring regularly for 4 minutes, or until they start to soften and turn translucent.

Spoon in the garlic and ginger puree and continue to fry for another minute, stirring regularly before pouring in the spice paste along with 50ml of water. Stir-fry for 2 minutes. If the mixture starts to burn or stick to the bottom of the pan then pour in another splash of water and reduce the heat a little.

Add the lamb chunks and fry, stirring for 1 minute. Pour in 250ml of stock or water and bring to the boil.

Put a lid on and simmer for 1 hour, until the meat is just tender. Keep checking on the curry during the cooking time and if you feel that too much liquid has been lost, add a little more. Give it a little stir every now and then to stop it from sticking to the bottom of the pan.

While the curry is cooking, make the cashew cream. Place the cashews into a bowl and cover them with boiling water. Leave them to sit for at least 30 minutes, then drain, discarding the water. Tip the cashews into a blender and blitz until smooth. Keep to one side until needed.

After 1 hour, when you are happy that the lamb is tender, stir in the cauliflower florets and lentils. You will have to prod them a little to cover them in the sauce, adding a little more water if needed. Simmer the curry uncovered for 25 minutes, or until the cauliflower is tender.

Stir in the cashew cream, spinach and chopped coriander, and then divide between your bowls or plates.

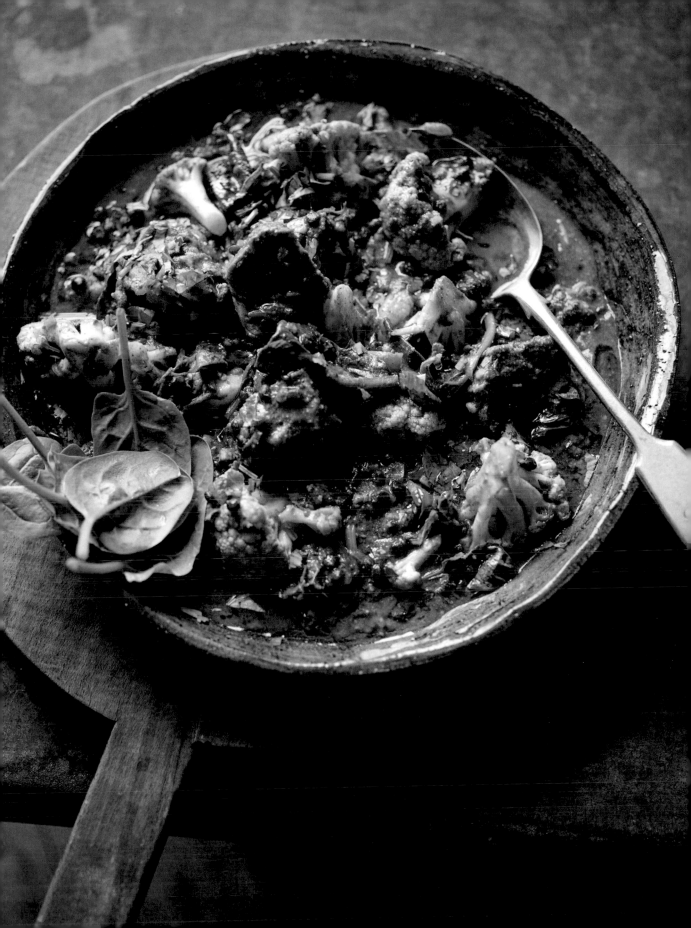

REDUCED-CARB

GOOEY GOAT'S CHEESE CHICKEN

Errm, chicken stuffed with goat's cheese and wrapped in bacon? Yes please. Sold. Don't be scared of the figs. They look weird but they taste awesome with the cheese.

◆PREP 15 MINS
◆COOK 20 MINS

4 skinless chicken breasts
150g soft goat's cheese
small bunch of chives, finely chopped
black pepper
12 rashers of unsmoked streaky bacon
6 ripe figs, cut into quarters
80g walnut pieces
1 red onion, finely sliced
4 large handfuls of rocket
drizzle of balsamic vinegar

Preheat your oven to 180°C (fan 160°C/gas mark 4).

Take one chicken breast and use a small knife to make a slit in the side of the thickest part, being careful not to cut all the way through to the other side. Repeat the process with the other chicken breasts.

Mix together the goat's cheese with the chives and season with black pepper.

Pick up a chicken breast and use a teaspoon to stuff a quarter of the goat's cheese mixture into the slit in the side – try to get as much in as possible. Wrap the stuffed chicken breast in three rashers of bacon and place it onto a roasting tray.

Repeat the process with the remaining chicken breasts, cheese and bacon. Slide the stuffed breasts into the oven and bake for 20 minutes, or until cooked. Check by slicing into one of the larger pieces to make sure the meat is white all the way through, with no raw pink bits left.

While the chicken is roasting, toss together all of the remaining ingredients and divide between four plates.

When you are happy that the chicken is cooked, remove it from the oven and leave to rest for a couple of minutes. Serve it on top of the salad and dive in.

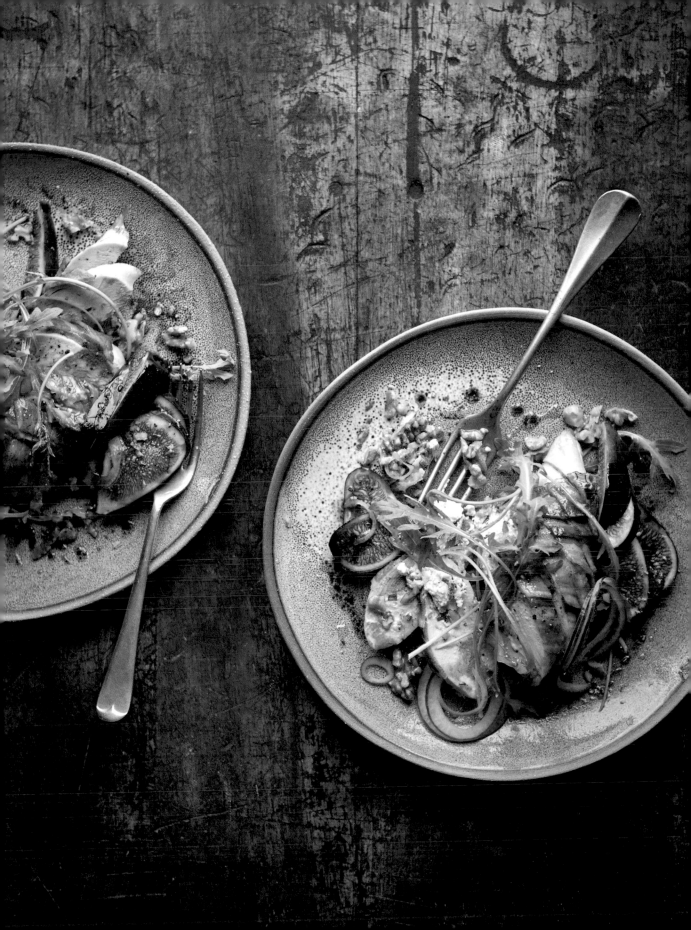

REDUCED-CARB
◆LOW & SLOW

CRISPY DUCK PANCAKES

Whenever I eat out with friends at a Chinese restaurant these pancakes are my go-to dish. I absolutely love them. You may not have cooked duck before but give it a go, it's easier than you think.

◆PREP 15 MINS,
 PLUS MARINATING TIME
◆COOK 1 HR 50 MINS

6 duck legs
250ml shaoxing wine
1 onion, roughly chopped
6 cloves garlic, bashed and
left whole
15cm orange peel
4 star anise
50g fresh ginger, roughly
chopped
500ml chicken stock
200ml hoisin sauce
6 spring onions, finely sliced
1 cucumber, de-seeded and cut
into 2.5cm batons
20–25 shop-bought Chinese-style
pancakes

Put the duck legs into the bottom of a large saucepan and pour over the shaoxing wine. Chuck in the chopped onion, garlic, orange peel, star anise and ginger and leave to sit for half an hour.

Pour over enough chicken stock to cover the legs and then put the pan on a high heat. Bring to the boil, and then simmer the legs for 1 hour 20 minutes, until incredibly tender. Remove the pan from the heat and leave the legs to cool completely in the cooking liquid.

Preheat your oven to 200°C (fan 180°C/gas mark 6).

Mix the hoisin sauce with about 3 tablespoons of the cooking liquid from the pan. Carefully lift the duck legs out of the liquid, pat dry with kitchen roll and then lay them in a large roasting tray. Pour the hoisin sauce mixture all over the legs, turning them to completely cover each leg. Slide the roasting tray into the oven and cook for 30 minutes, turning the legs halfway through.

While the legs are roasting, lay out the spring onions and cucumber and heat the pancakes, either in a steamer or in the microwave.

When the legs are ready, transfer them from the tray onto a plate, scraping out as much of the sauce as possible. Break up the tender meat with a couple of forks and start building your pancakes.

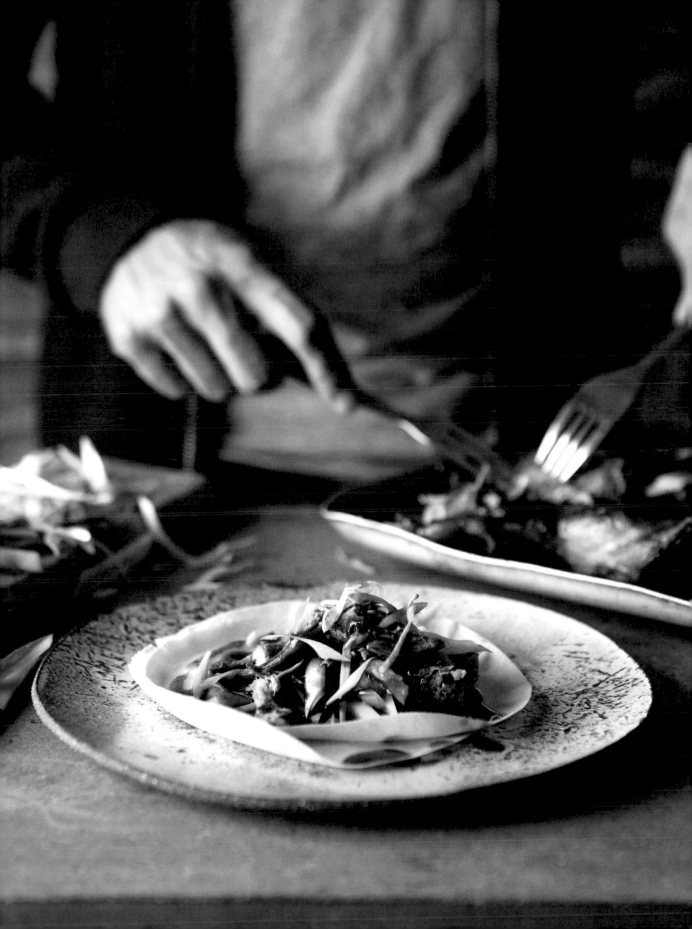

REDUCED-CARB

GRILLED SEA BASS WITH CAVOLO NERO

You may not have heard of cavolo nero before. It's similar to kale, really good for you and you can find it in most supermarkets. Be sure to grill your sea bass skin-side up so it's nice and crispy.

◆PREP 15 MINS
◆COOK 25 MINS

2 fennel bulbs, cut lengthways into 1cm strips

1 tsp chilli flakes

1 tsp fennel seeds

juice of 1 lemon

1½ tbsp fish sauce

250g cavolo nero, thick stalks removed and leaves cut roughly into thirds

75g hazelnuts

8 x 100–125g sea bass fillets, skin-on

2 tsp olive oil

salt

small bunch of parsley, roughly chopped, to serve

Preheat your oven to 190°C (fan 170°C/gas mark 5).

Line a baking tray with a large piece of tin foil and place the slices of fennel in the middle. Sprinkle with the chilli flakes and fennel seeds and then pour over the lemon juice and fish sauce along with 2 tablespoons of water. Wrap up the sides to create a parcel. Slide the tray into the oven and bake for 10 minutes, until the fennel is so soft that you can push a knife through it.

Carefully open up the parcel and add the cavolo nero and hazelnuts. Pour in another tablespoon of water, rewrap the parcel and slide it back into the oven for a final 10 minutes.

Line another baking tray with greaseproof paper. Turn your grill on to maximum and lay the sea bass fillets, skin-side up, on the lined baking tray. Drizzle the fillets with the oil, season with salt and grill for 6 minutes without turning them, until the skin crisps up and the flesh is cooked all the way through.

When the vegetables have had their cooking time, remove them from the oven and carefully open up the parcel again, making sure you dodge the escaping hot steam. Stir the chopped parsley through the vegetables and then plate up.

Top the vegetables with two fillets of fish per person and serve.

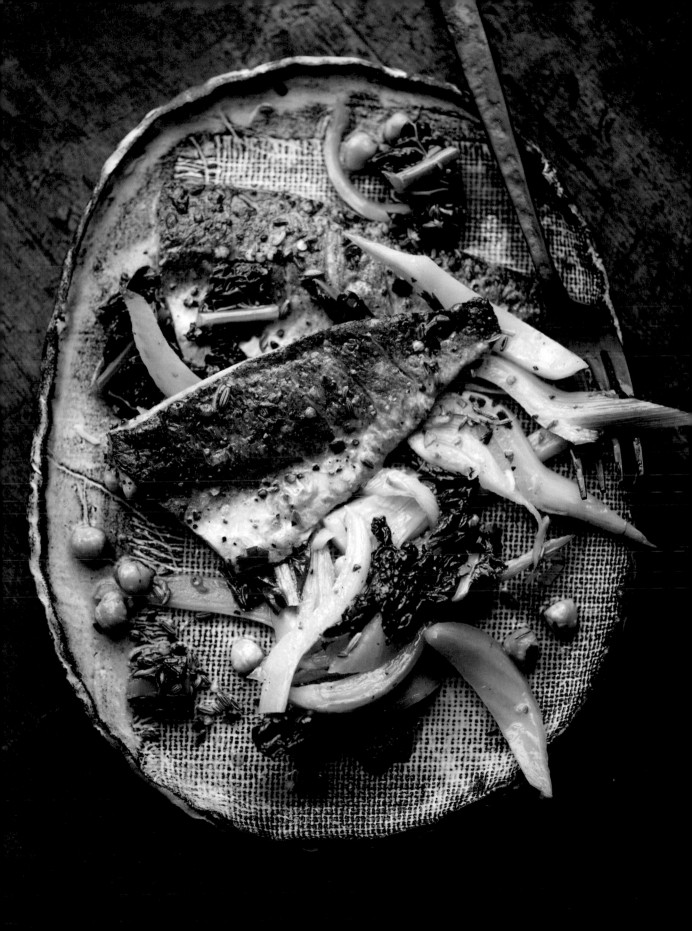

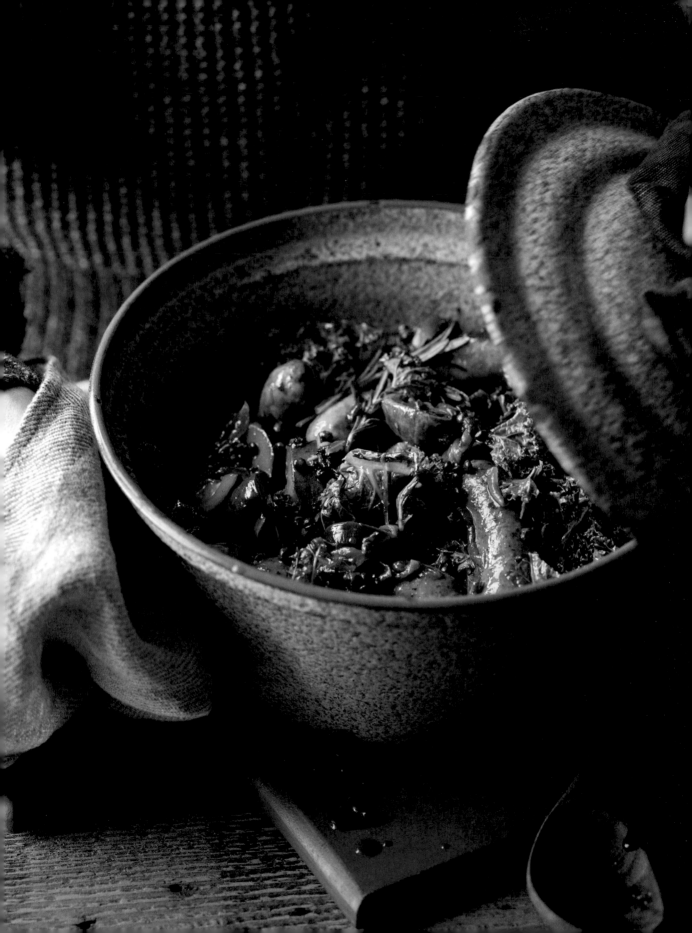

REDUCED-CARB

SAUSAGE & RED WINE CASSEROLE

This is a really hearty dish for cosy family nights in. It's a one-pot wonder and full of flavour – you'll definitely want to make this one again.

➡PREP 10 MINS
➡COOK 45 MINS

½ tbsp coconut oil

12 sausages

2 red onions, sliced

3 cloves garlic, bashed and left whole

2 large sprigs of rosemary

400g chestnut mushrooms, roughly halved

1 courgette, cut into 2cm chunks

200ml red wine

200ml chicken stock

125g ready-to-eat lentils

4 large handfuls of kale, stalks removed

Melt the oil in a large saucepan over a medium heat. When it is hot, carefully lay in the sausages and slowly brown all over – frying them too quickly often makes them burst. When the sausages are browned all over, remove them to a plate.

Slide the sliced onions into the saucepan along with the garlic and the sprigs of rosemary. Fry, stirring every now and then for 3 minutes, or until the onion is beginning to soften. Increase the heat to medium-high and chuck in the mushrooms and courgette, tossing them in the rest of the mixture. Fry everything together for 3 minutes, then return the sausages to the pan.

Crank up the heat to maximum and when everything in the pan is sizzling, pour in the red wine and let it bubble away until it has reduced by a third. Pour in the chicken stock and bring it to a simmer. Cook uncovered for 25 minutes, or until you are happy that the sausages are fully cooked through – check by cutting into one to make sure there is no raw pink meat left.

Add the lentils and kale, prodding and stirring them with a wooden spoon. Keep cooking the casserole for about 5 minutes, or until the kale is cooked to your liking. Serve up and tuck in.

REDUCED-CARB

SALMON & RED PEPPER STEW

Minimal prep time, maximum flavour: this is a winner all year round.

◆PREP 12 MINS
◆COOK 1 HR

2 tbsp olive oil
1 red onion, sliced
2 red peppers, finely sliced
1 yellow pepper, finely sliced
1 courgette, diced
1 bay leaf
3 sprigs of thyme
2½ tbsp tomato puree
1 tbsp sherry vinegar
6 x 125g skinless salmon fillets
salt and pepper

To serve
bunch of basil, leaves only
1 lemon, cut into wedges – optional

Equipment
large ovenproof saucepan or hob-proof casserole dish

Heat the olive oil in a large ovenproof saucepan or hob-proof casserole dish over a medium to high heat. When it is hot, add the red onion, peppers and courgette. Fry, stirring regularly for about 5 minutes, or until the vegetables are starting to soften.

Add the bay leaf, thyme sprigs and tomato puree, and continue to fry, stirring almost constantly for 2 minutes, until the puree darkens significantly in colour. Pour in the vinegar and let it bubble up and pretty much completely evaporate.

Pour in 500ml of water and bring to a simmer. Cook the pepper stew like this for about 45 minutes, or until the peppers are very soft. Add more water if you think it needs it.

Preheat your oven to 190°C (fan 170°C/gas mark 5).

When the peppers are nicely soft, nestle the salmon fillets in the mixture and season with salt and pepper. Slide the whole uncovered pan into the oven and bake for 12 minutes, or until the salmon is just cooked through – you can check this by slicing into the thick end of a fillet to make sure the flesh has turned matt pink.

When the fish is cooked, sprinkle over the basil leaves, top with lemon wedges, if you like, and serve.

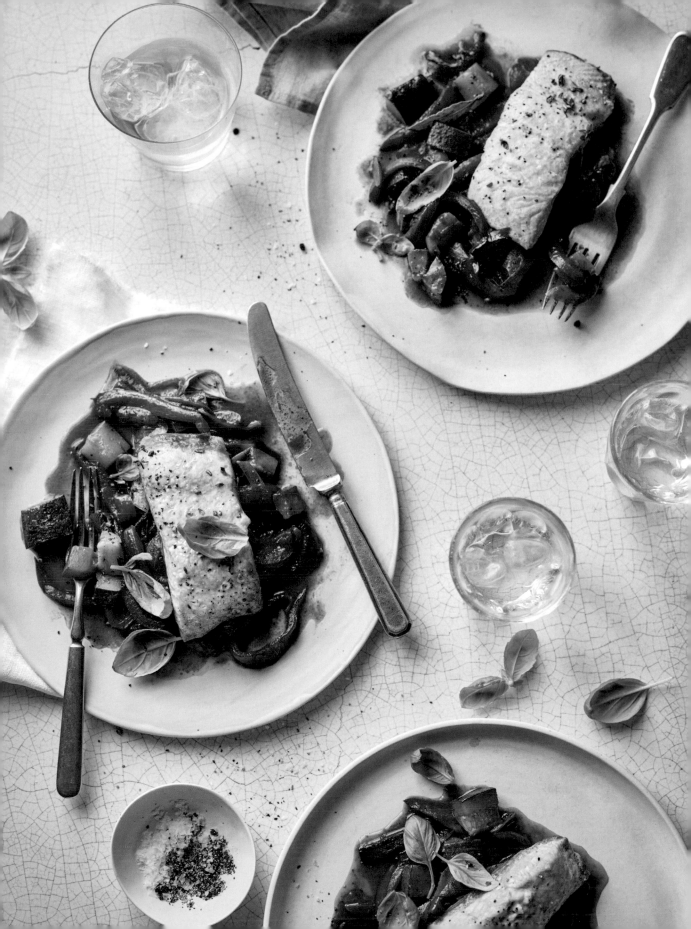

STEAK AT-A-GLANCE

I'm going to be honest with you, it's taken me ages to learn how to cook a good steak. I've burned a fair few in my time but I've finally nailed it and I'm going to share my top tips with you now. I recommend visiting your local butcher who can give you a steer on the different types of cuts.

COOK YOUR STEAK LIKE A BOSS

Take the steak out of the fridge about an hour in advance of serving. Cover the meat loosely with cling film and leave it to come to room temperature – this allows the steak to cook evenly and more quickly. If you're planning to rest the cooked steaks in the oven (see below), then preheat your oven to its lowest setting.

Open your windows or turn on the extractor fan, because steak cooking needs a very hot pan, which can smoke.

Rub each steak all over with olive oil and season generously with salt and pepper. Place a heavy-based pan or griddle pan over a medium heat. If you're cooking fillet steaks, it is best to finish them in the oven, so choose an ovenproof frying pan.

When your pan is smoking hot, carefully lay two steaks at a time into your pan and fry them hard. Flip them over every minute until they are cooked to your liking (see timings, right).

Rest the steaks – this is perhaps the most important part of the cooking process as it helps the steak to cook evenly and also tenderizes the meat. Rest your steak for at least half the cooking time, or ideally for the whole cooking time. The best place to rest steaks is on a plate in your preheated oven, covered loosely with tin foil. Repeat the process with the remaining steaks. Perfection.

TIMINGS

These timings are accurate for 3–3.5cm-thick steaks, cooked from room temperature.

Rare (top right)
1 minute on each side, then 30 seconds on each side.

Medium rare (middle right)
1 minute on each side, then another minute on each side, then 30 seconds on each side.

Well done (bottom right)
1 minute on each side, then another minute on each side, then a third minute on each side, then 30 seconds on each side.

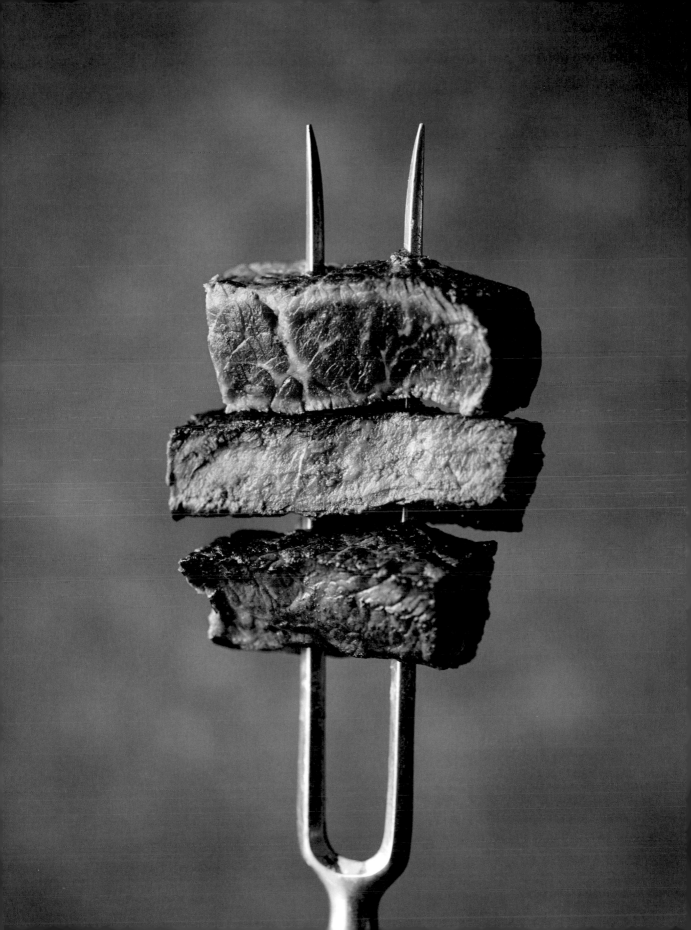

CHOOSE YOUR STEAK

RIB-EYE

This cut has become increasingly popular over the last few years because of the flavour–price ratio. Rib-eye is cheaper than sirloin and fillet, but delivers on flavour and texture because it has a good level of fat in the meat. Because of the fat content, rib-eye is best eaten as part of a reduced-carb meal, and cooked to medium rare.

FILLET

The most expensive and luxurious of all steaks, fillet is meltingly tender. I would reserve this for loved ones on very special occasions. Because of the low fat content it is best enjoyed rare – there is no point cooking it beyond medium rare. It's a great cut of meat for post-workout meals, but you could also cook it with a lump of butter for a reduced-carb meal.

SIRLOIN

This is a real all-rounder. It is one of the pricier steaks, but for good reason, because it has a decent level of fat and so has both great flavour and texture. This is the steak to cook if you want to please everybody. Use sirloin for reduced-carb recipes, or trim off the visible fat and serve as a post-workout meal.

RUMP

There isn't a lot of fat in rump steak apart from what's visible, so it is perfect for post-workout meals. It is the cheapest of the steaks as well so won't break the bank. Because of its lean nature, quick cooking is best: I recommend rare to medium rare.

REDUCED-CARB

BEARNAISE SAUCE

This sauce comes all the way from classic French kitchens. To make clarified butter, simply melt a load of butter and skim the nasty solid stuff from the surface. Pour the clear clarified butter out of the pan into a jug, leaving the solids at the bottom of the pan, which you can discard.

→PREP 15 MINS
→COOK 5 MINS

60ml white wine vinegar
2 large shallots, diced
5 sprigs of tarragon
2 egg yolks
180g clarified butter (from melting 250g butter)

Place the vinegar, shallots and 3 sprigs of tarragon into a small saucepan and bring to the boil. Simmer until the liquid has reduced by about three-quarters and about a tablespoon of vinegar is left. Strain into a large heatproof bowl and leave to cool.

Bring a pan of water to the boil. Drop the egg yolks into the vinegar and whisk together. Place the bowl over the saucepan of boiling water, making sure the surface of the water doesn't come into contact with the base of the bowl.

Whisk the yolks and vinegar together for a further 5 minutes over the hot pan of water. The mixture will increase in volume, thicken and turn pale. Remove the bowl from the top of the pan.

This next bit is probably a job for two people: while constantly whisking, drizzle in the clarified butter, starting slowly then gradually increasing the speed as more butter is incorporated and the mixture thickens. Do not pour in too much butter at once or the sauce will split.

When you have whisked in all the butter, add 2–3 tablespoons of warm water to the mixture to loosen it to a thick pouring consistency.

Chop up the leaves from the remaining 2 sprigs of tarragon. Stir it through your béarnaise sauce and serve immediately with the cooked steak.

SEE PHOTO ON PAGE 57 ➡

SERVES 4

REDUCED-CARB

PINK PEPPERCORN SAUCE

This is the classic sauce to accompany steak. I recommend pink or even green peppercorns, not just for how they look, but also because they have a softer flavour than black peppercorns. Brandy is delicious and traditional, but leave it out if you prefer.

◆PREP 5 MINS
◆COOK 15 MINS

knob of butter
1 onion, diced
2 sprigs of thyme
500ml chicken stock,
fresh if possible
200ml double cream
capful of brandy – optional
20g pink peppercorns
salt

Melt the butter in a medium saucepan over a medium to high heat. When it is bubbling, slide in the chopped onion and cook, stirring regularly for 4 minutes.

Add the sprigs of thyme and fry, stirring regularly for a further 3 minutes.

Crank up the heat to maximum and pour in the chicken stock. Boil the stock until it has reduced by half and then pour in the cream and boil until reduced by half again. Strain the sauce into a jug, and discard the onion and thyme.

Return the sauce to the saucepan over a low heat. Add the capful of brandy, if using, and the pink peppercorns, then bring to the boil one last time. Simmer for 5 minutes, season with salt and serve.

★ *FOR THE TASTIEST RESULTS, USE FRESH STOCK RATHER THAN STOCK CUBES.*

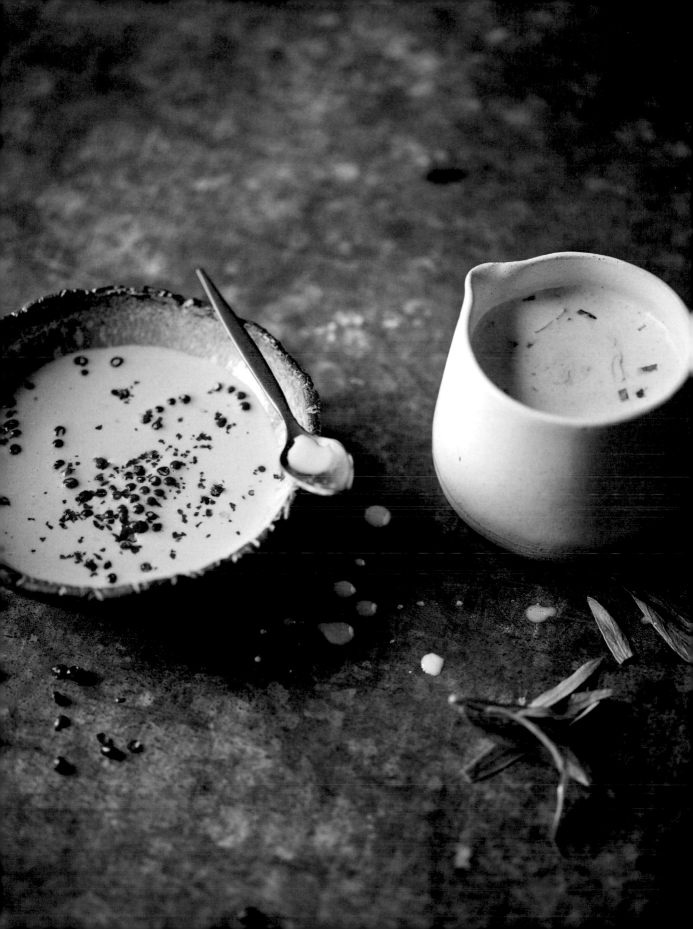

Serves 4

REDUCED-CARB

LOW-CARB BANGERS & MASH

This is a really awesome low-carb alternative to potato mash, perfect for rest days. The kids probably won't even realize they're eating a load of cauliflower, LOL. It's so tasty I reckon you'll want this cheesy alternative every time. Serve it up with the sage and onion gravy from my Toad in the hole (see page 79).

→PREP 15 MINS
→COOK 20 MINS

1 medium cauliflower, florets only (about 600g)
1 x 400g tin of butter beans, drained and rinsed (about 240g)
12 sausages
25g parmesan, grated
40g cheddar, grated
salt and pepper

To serve
sage and onion gravy (see page 79)
small bunch of parsley, finely chopped
steamed greens

Preheat your grill to maximum.

Bring a large pan of water to the boil and then chuck in the cauliflower florets and the drained butter beans. Simmer for 15 minutes, or until soft. Drain the cauliflower and beans thoroughly and return to the warm pan.

While the cauliflower and beans are simmering away, slide the sausages under the grill and cook them for about 12 minutes, turning a couple of times until they are cooked through.

While the cauliflower and beans are hot, roughly mash the whole lot together (you won't end up with a smooth mash; it will still have texture to it). Add both kinds of cheese and stir in to melt. Add a little salt and pepper if you think it needs it.

By now your sausages should be cooked, so serve up the cheesy mash with three sausages each and a ladleful of sage and onion gravy. Sprinkle with chopped parsley and serve with a healthy portion of steamed greens on the side.

★ *I LIKE A STRAIGHT-UP PORK BANGER FOR THIS CLASSIC, BUT GO FOR WHAT YOU LIKE.*

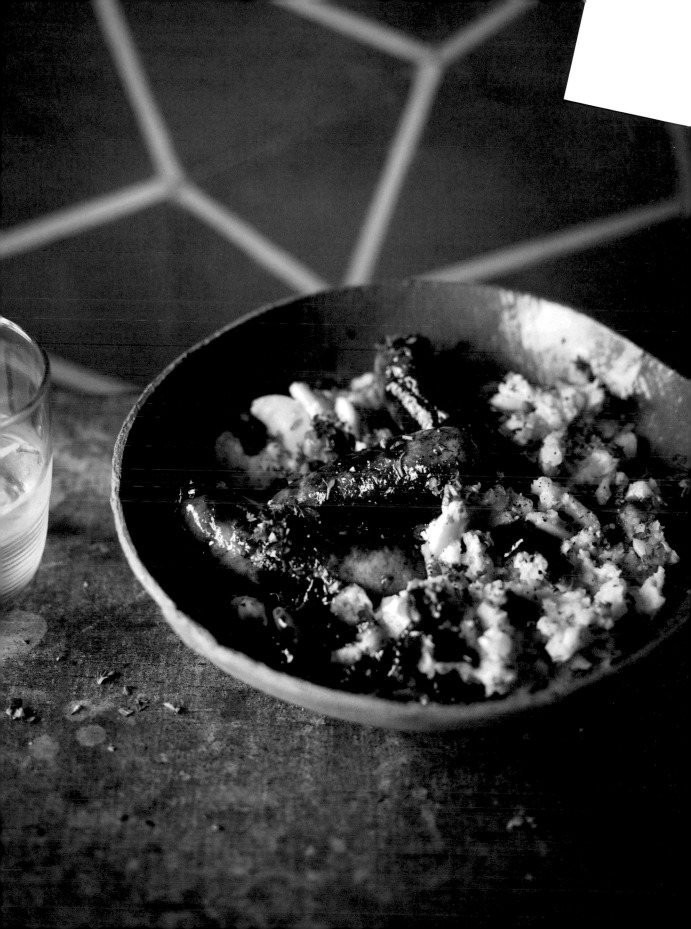

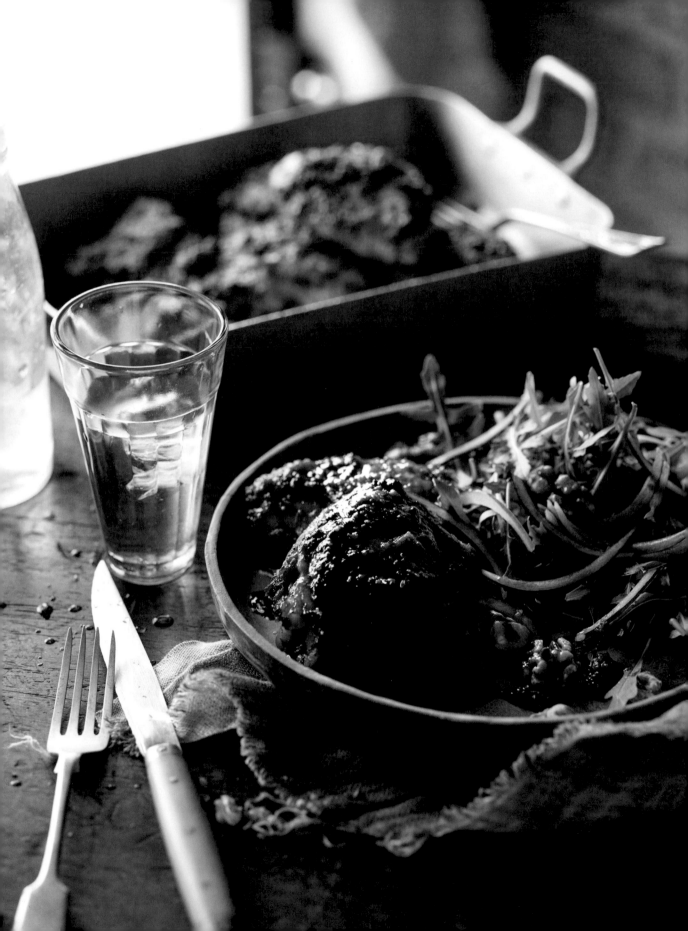

REDUCED-CARB

MEXICAN CHICKEN TRAY BAKE

The flavours in this are really going to knock your socks off! It takes very little prep time so give it a go. You won't be disappointed.

➤**PREP 12 MINS**
➤**COOK 50 MINS**

8 chicken leg-and-thigh portions, bone-in and skin-on
2 red onions
4 cloves garlic, roughly chopped
1 red pepper, roughly chopped
3 tbsp chipotle paste
juice of 1 orange
1 tbsp olive oil
1 tbsp sundried tomato paste
salt and pepper
juice of 2 limes

To serve
4 large handfuls of rocket
50g walnuts, roughly chopped

Equipment
blender

Preheat your oven to 180°C (fan 160°C/gas mark 4).

Using a sharp knife, slash the skin of each piece of chicken in a few places – this helps the chipotle mixture to flavour the chicken. Lay the slashed chicken pieces in a roasting tray.

Roughly chop one of the red onions and add it to a blender. Add the garlic, red pepper, chipotle paste, orange juice, olive oil and sundried tomato paste along with a good pinch of salt and pepper. Blitz until smooth, adding a little splash of warm water if you have trouble getting it started.

Pour the mixture all over the chicken pieces, making sure it covers both sides and you work it into the slashes in the chicken skin. Slide the tray into the oven and roast for 50 minutes.

While the chicken is cooking, finely slice the second red onion and put it into a bowl with the lime juice. Leave the onion sitting in the juice until you are ready to serve – this process softens the taste of raw onion.

Check the chicken is cooked by slicing into one of the larger pieces to make sure the meat is white all the way through, with no raw pink bits left.

Allow the cooked chicken to rest for 5 minutes, then load it up on plates and top with the lime-soaked red onion, rocket and chopped walnuts.

Serves 4

REDUCED-CARB

CREAMY PARMESAN PESTO CHICKEN

Here's a proper tasty, comforting dish for the family that everyone will love. I've given you a recipe to make your own pesto, but you can also use a shop-bought one to make life even easier.

➤ PREP 15 MINS
➤ COOK 25 MINS

1½ tbsp coconut oil

4 chicken breasts, skin-on

2 large bunches of basil, thick stalks removed

2 cloves garlic, roughly chopped

30g pine nuts

65g parmesan, grated

zest of 1 lemon

50ml olive oil

salt and pepper

1 onion, diced

3 rashers of smoked streaky bacon, cut into 1cm strips

2 carrots, diced

2 celery sticks, diced

50ml chicken stock

80g mascarpone

1 bunch of chives, finely sliced

steamed midget trees (tender-stem broccoli) or kale, to serve

Equipment
food processor

Melt half of the coconut oil in a large frying pan over a medium heat. When it is hot, carefully lay the chicken breasts into the pan, skin-side down, and leave to cook over the medium heat for about 10 minutes, or until the skin has turned golden.

While the chicken is cooking, make the pesto by placing the basil, garlic, pine nuts, 50g of the parmesan, lemon zest, olive oil and 50ml of warm water into a food processor along with a generous pinch of salt and pepper. Blitz until smooth, adding a little more water if it needs helping along. Keep the pesto to one side.

After 10 minutes in the frying pan, the chicken skin should be beautifully golden and some of the fat rendered out of the skin. Transfer the breasts to a plate and add the remaining coconut oil, onion, bacon, carrots and celery, and sweat them over a medium to high heat for 5 minutes, or until they are just beginning to soften.

Lay the chicken breasts back into the pan, flesh-side down, and pour in the chicken stock. Let it bubble and simmer for 2–3 minutes, or until you are happy that the chicken is cooked through. Check by slicing into one of the larger pieces to make sure the meat is white all the way through, with no raw pink bits left. Stir in the mascarpone to make a creamy sauce, then spoon in the pesto and stir until totally combined.

Take the pan off the heat and sprinkle in the remaining parmesan and the chives. Serve with steamed midget trees or kale.

REDUCED-CARB
→MAKE AHEAD

→PREP 15 MINS
→COOK 50 MINS

2 knobs of butter
1 red onion, diced
4 skinless chicken breasts,
cut into 2cm slices
450g baby spinach
200g feta
20g dill, finely chopped
2 tbsp pine nuts
salt and pepper
4 large sheets of filo pastry
green salad, to serve

Equipment
23cm springform cake tin

CHICKEN & FETA FILO PIE

If you enjoyed 'Joe's chicken pie' from my first book then you'll love this one. It also tastes great at room temperature the next day, so could make an ideal lunch for work.

Preheat your oven to 180°C (fan 160°C/gas mark 4).

Melt a knob of butter in a large frying pan over a medium to high heat. When it is hot, slide in the onion and fry for 2 minutes. Add the chicken to the frying pan and cook for about 4 minutes or until the chicken is just cooked through.

Pile the spinach into the pan and allow it to wilt. Tip the mixture into a bowl and add the feta, dill and pine nuts. Season with salt and pepper and leave the mixture to cool to room temperature.

Melt the second knob of butter in a small saucepan. Use a pastry brush to splash some of the melted butter all around the base and sides of the cake tin.

Drape one sheet of the filo pastry over the cake tin and ease it down so that it covers the base of the tin. Lightly push it against the sides so that it sticks, but drapes over the sides.

Brush the filo with a little melted butter and then lay a second sheet on top, at a 45-degree angle to the first. Brush again with a little more melted butter. Lay your third sheet of filo at a 45-degree angle to the second – this ensures that the base and sides are fully covered.

Over the sink, give the chicken mixture a little squeeze with the back of a wooden spoon to remove excess liquid. Pile the mixture into the lined tin, flattening it out with the spoon.

Scrunch up your final sheet of filo and place it on top of the mixture, then fold the overhanging pastry over the mixture so that the filling is totally covered. Drizzle over any leftover melted butter and slide the tin into the oven. Bake for 40 minutes.

When the pie is baked, take it from the oven and leave to rest for 10 minutes, then carefully release from the tin, slide onto a plate and enjoy with a big green salad.

REDUCED-CARB

THE BODY COACH ROAST BEEF

I love a good roast and this one has all the trimmings, including swede mash and cauliflower cheese. There are no Yorkshire puddings I'm afraid but it tastes lovely and will keep you lean.

➡ **PREP 20 MINS**
➡ **COOK 45 MINS**

1.5kg piece of sirloin, at room temperature
salt and pepper
4 carrots, roughly chopped
1 large swede, roughly cubed
2 heads of cauliflower, florets only (about 650g)
215g mascarpone
1 egg
2 spring onions, finely sliced
1 tsp English mustard
40g cheddar, grated
25g parmesan, grated
20g butter
1 bay leaf
2 sprigs of thyme
1 tbsp plain flour
500ml good-quality beef stock

To serve
small bunch of parsley, finely chopped
steamed greens

Preheat your oven to 220°C (fan 200°C/gas mark 7).

Season the beef with salt and pepper and place it onto a roasting tin. Slide it into the oven and roast for 15 minutes. Reduce the temperature to 175°C (fan 155°C/gas mark 4) and continue to roast the beef for 25 minutes. Remove it from the oven, wrap it tightly in tin foil and leave it to rest on a plate for at least 20 minutes. Do not throw away the fat and cooking juices from the tin.

While the beef is roasting, bring two large saucepans of water to the boil. Chuck the carrots and swede into one of the pans and simmer for about 20 minutes, or until they are totally tender.

Drop the cauliflower florets into the other pan and simmer for about 8 minutes, or until the florets are just tender. Drain the florets in a sieve or colander and leave to steam dry.

Beat together the mascarpone, egg, spring onions and mustard along with a good pinch of salt and pepper. The mascarpone should loosen as you beat it, but if not, add a splash of water until the mixture reaches 'dolloping' consistency.

Pile the cauliflower florets into an oven dish and scrape the mascarpone mixture over the top, spreading it out. Scatter the cheddar and parmesan over the top of the dish and then slide the cauliflower into the oven and bake for 25 minutes, or until the mascarpone is bubbling and the cheese has browned. ➡

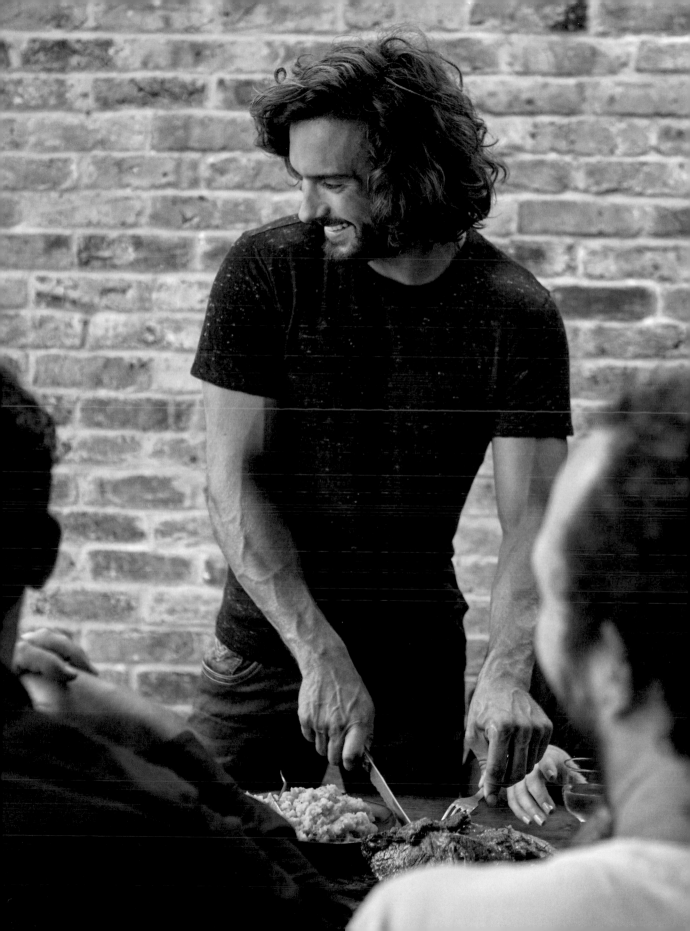

THE BODY COACH
ROAST BEEF (CONTINUED)

When the swede and carrots are tender, thoroughly drain them in a sieve or colander and tip them back into the pan along with the butter. Add a bit of salt and a generous pinch of pepper and mash the lot together – you don't want to mash it up too much as a bit of texture is nice. Keep warm until you're ready to serve.

Place the roasting tin over a low to medium heat (or pour the beef fat into a small pan if you don't have a hob-proof roasting tin). Add the bay leaf and sprigs of thyme, sprinkle in the flour and stir to combine with the juices to form a smooth paste. Cook the paste for about 1 minute then start gradually adding in the beef stock – if you pour too much in too quickly then you will end up with lumpy gravy.

Keep stirring in the beef stock until it has all been incorporated, then bring to the boil and remove from the heat. Scatter with chopped parsley and serve up the roast beef dinner with some freshly steamed greens.

★ *IF YOU STEAM OR BOIL GREENS TO GO ON THE SIDE, TRY SAVING THE COOKING LIQUID AND USING IT TO MAKE YOUR STOCK FOR THE GRAVY.*

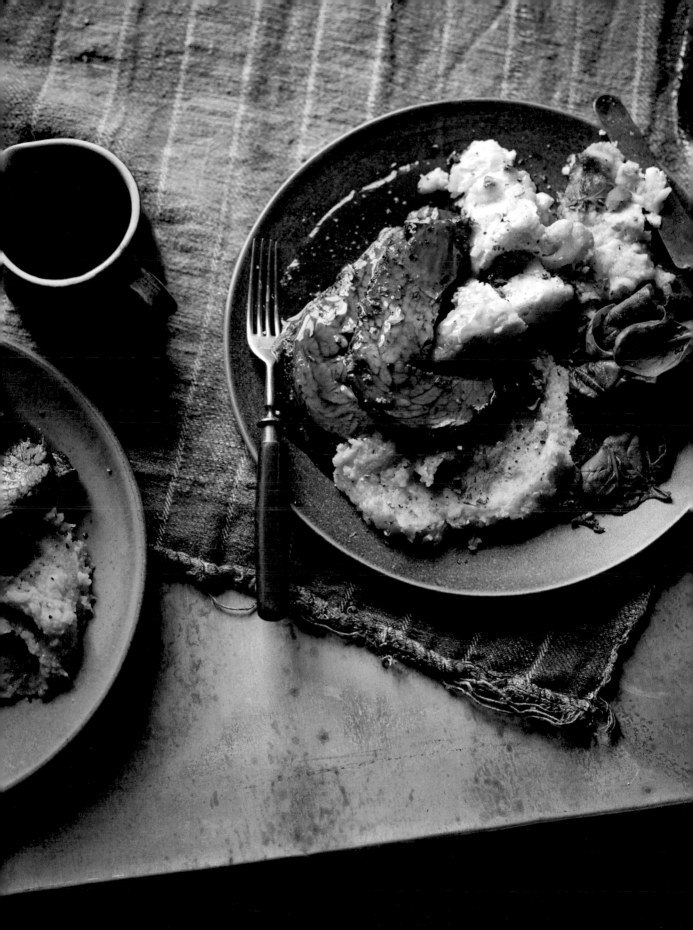

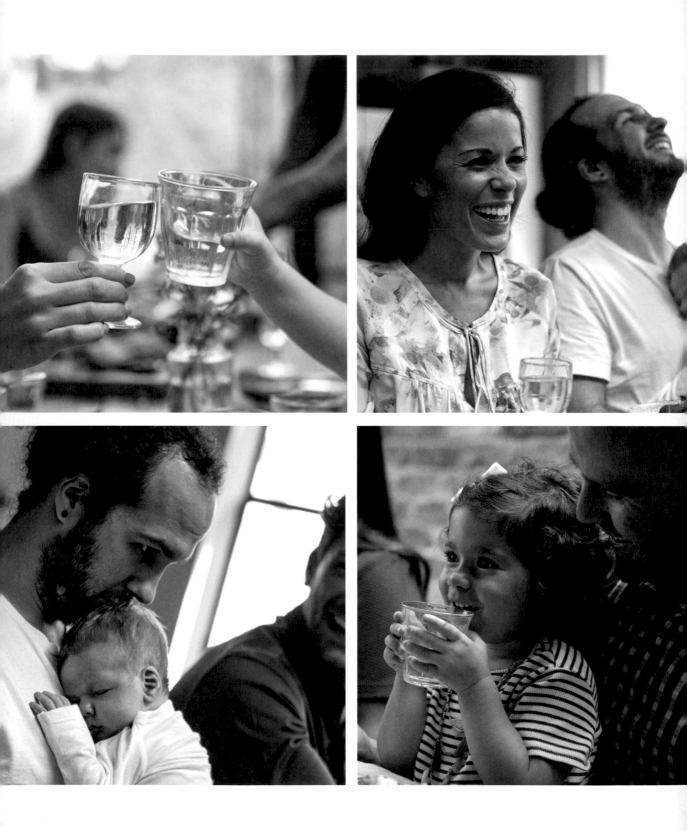

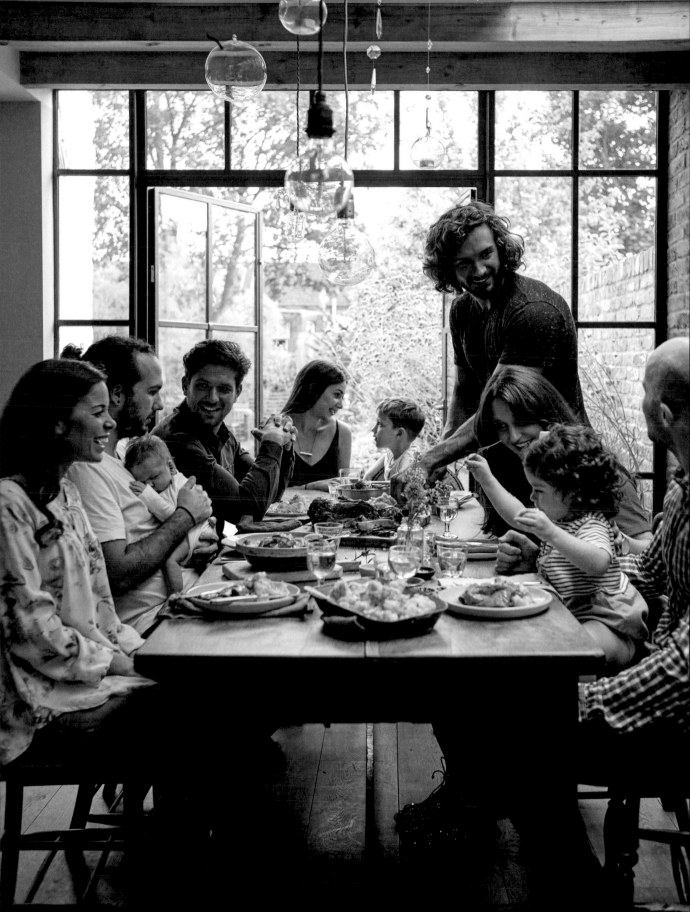

REDUCED-CARB

JOE'S FISH PIE

After the success of 'Joe's chicken pie' in my first book I decided to create an even tastier one. This pie uses smoked haddock, salmon and prawns and it tastes unbelievable. It's so creamy inside and the crispy filo pastry on top just seals the deal for me.

➧**PREP 15 MINS**
➧**COOK 30 MINS**

4 eggs
large knob of butter
1 onion, diced
¼ tsp ground mace
1 bay leaf
180g skinless smoked haddock, cut into 3cm chunks
200ml fish stock
75ml double cream
400g skinless salmon, cut into 3cm chunks
180g raw king prawns, peeled
50g parmesan, grated
½ bunch of parsley, finely chopped
3 large sheets of filo pastry (1 x 270g pack)
steamed greens or salad, to serve

Equipment
23 x 18cm baking dish

Preheat your oven to 180°C (fan 160°C/gas mark 4) and bring a medium saucepan of water to the boil.

Gently lower in the eggs and simmer for 8 minutes. When they are cooked, run them under cold water and peel each one. Set the eggs to one side.

While the eggs are cooking, melt the butter in a saucepan over a medium to high heat. When it is bubbling, add the onion and cook for 3 minutes, or until the onion is beginning to soften.

Increase the heat to maximum and add the mace, bay leaf and haddock chunks. Fry the whole lot together for 1 minute and then pour in the stock. Bring to the boil and simmer for 1 minute, then add the double cream and bring to a simmer one last time before turning off the heat.

Add the salmon, prawns, parmesan and parsley and gently stir to combine everything. Roughly chop the boiled eggs and fold them through the mixture. Tip the whole lot into the baking dish.

Roughly scrunch up the filo pastry sheets and sit them on top of the mixture. Slide the fish pie into the oven and bake for 15 minutes, or until the pastry has coloured and the mixture is piping hot. Serve with steamed greens or a simple salad.

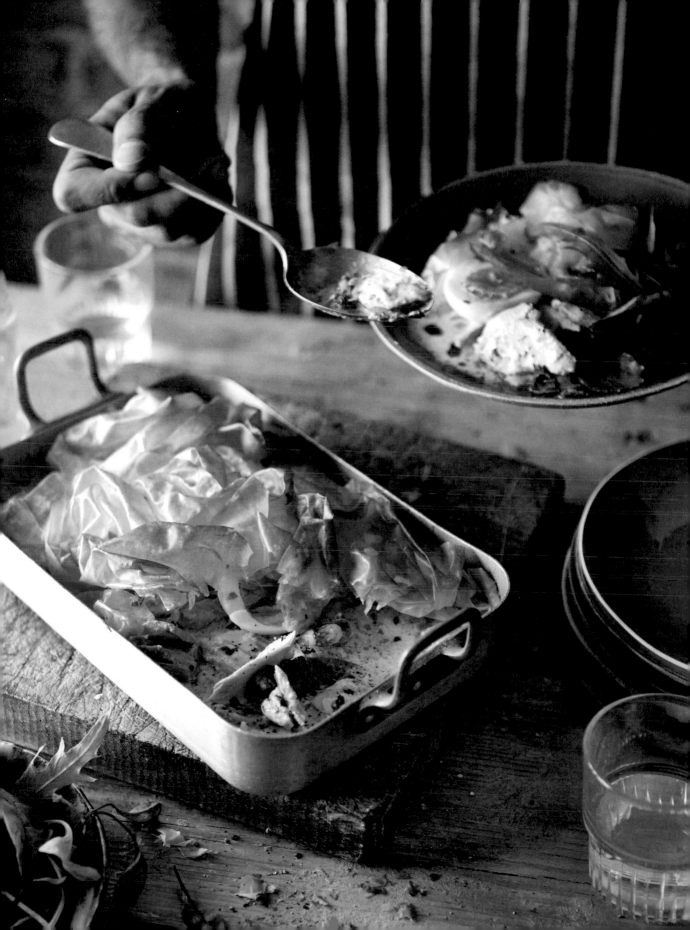

REDUCED-CARB

TUNA WITH SUNDRIED TOMATO TAPENADE

Tapenade is just a fancy word for blitzed-up black olives. This recipe makes more than you need, but you could eat the rest with some meat or chicken. Just keep the leftovers in a sealed container in the fridge for up to 4 days.

➔PREP 15 MINS
➔COOK 8 MINS

150g pitted black olives, roughly chopped

2 tbsp sundried tomato paste

1 small clove garlic, roughly chopped

½ bunch of basil, leaves only, roughly chopped

olive oil, for drizzling

2 eggs

125g midget trees (tender-stem broccoli), thick stalks cut in half lengthways

2 x 200g tuna steaks

salt and pepper

1 avocado, de-stoned and cut into thick wedges

handful of rocket

To serve
15g pumpkin seeds
1 lemon, cut into wedges

Equipment
blender

Bring a medium saucepan of water to the boil.

Place the olives, sundried tomato paste, garlic and basil into a blender and blitz until pretty smooth. It might be necessary to pour in a little drizzle of oil or water to get the blending started. Set aside your tapenade.

When the water is boiling, carefully lower in the eggs and boil for 7 minutes. When you have 2 minutes of cooking time left, add the midget trees to the saucepan. Drain the eggs and broccoli together in a sieve or colander and rinse both under cold running water. Set aside.

Heat a frying pan or griddle pan over a high heat. Drizzle a little olive oil over both sides of the tuna steaks and then season with salt and pepper. When your pan is very hot, carefully slide the tuna steaks in and cook for 2 minutes on each side.

Place the tuna on two plates and leave them to rest. Make a small salad with the midget trees, avocado and rocket, and pile it onto the plates with the tuna. Peel the eggs, cut them in half and then place them alongside. Finish your tasty meal with a scattering of pumpkin seeds, a dollop of the tapenade and a wedge of lemon.

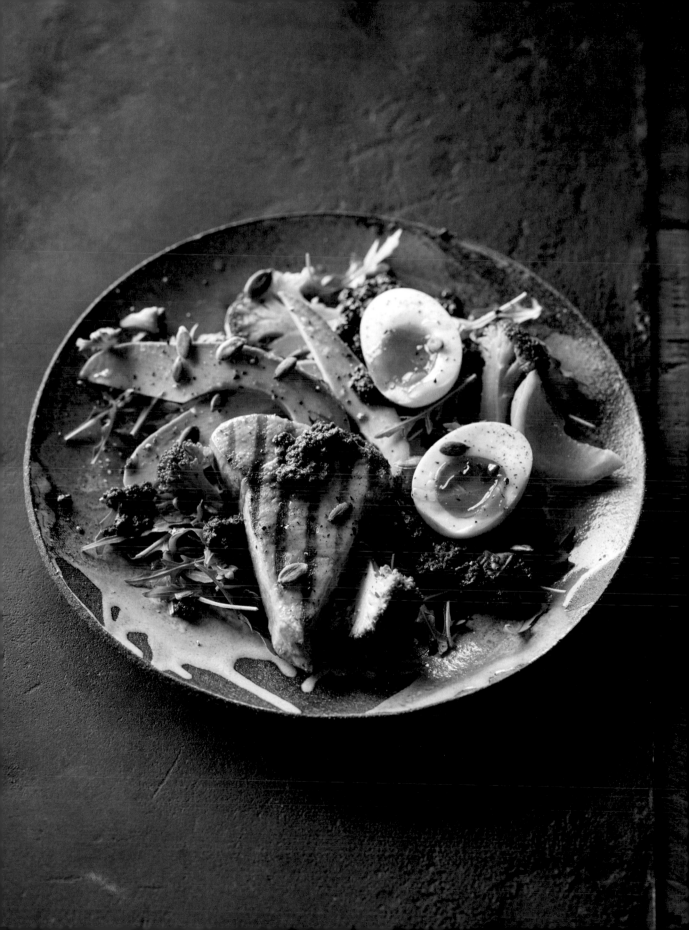

REDUCED-CARB

CHEESY ROAST SPATCHCOCK CHICKEN

You might not have spatchcocked a chicken before, but don't worry because it's really easy to do. It makes good use of a whole chicken and is much cheaper than buying chicken breasts on their own.

➧**PREP 15 MINS**
➧**COOK 1 HR**

1 whole chicken (about 1.5kg)
2 red onions, roughly cut into 8 wedges
3 courgettes, cut on the diagonal into 2.5cm chunks
3 sprigs of thyme
2 tsp olive oil
salt and pepper
1 tsp of dried oregano
1 x 400g tin chopped tomatoes
1 tbsp capers
16 pitted green olives
large bunch of basil, leaves only, roughly chopped, plus extra for garnish
175g ready-to-eat lentils
1 x 125g ball of mozzarella, squeezed to remove as much liquid as possible
rocket salad, to serve

Preheat your oven to 190°C (fan 170°C/gas mark 5).

To spatchcock your chicken, turn it upside down. Using a clean and sharp pair of scissors, cut either side of the backbone and then completely remove it. Turn the chicken over and then put your hands on top. Lean on the chicken to squash it down – at this point it may make a bone-cracking noise, but that's okay.

Chuck the red onion and courgette chunks into a medium roasting tray. Add the thyme and toss the ingredients together. Place the prepped chicken directly on top of the vegetables, drizzle with the olive oil, season with salt and pepper and then sprinkle with the dried oregano.

Slide the chicken into the oven and roast for 30 minutes.

While the chicken is cooking, mix together the chopped tomatoes, capers, green olives, chopped basil and lentils, along with 50ml of water and a good pinch of salt and pepper.

When the chicken has been cooking for 30 minutes, remove the tray from the oven and pour in the tomato mixture, lifting the chicken a little so that the mixture combines with the roasting vegetables underneath. Slide the tray back into the oven, reduce the temperature to 180°C (fan 160°C/gas mark 4) and roast for a further 15 minutes.

Remove the tray from the oven, tear up the mozzarella and dot all around in the tomato sauce. Slide the tray back into the oven and roast for a final 10–15 minutes, by which time the chicken will be cooked through and the mozzarella bubbling.

Top your roast with the remaining basil and serve with a generous rocket salad.

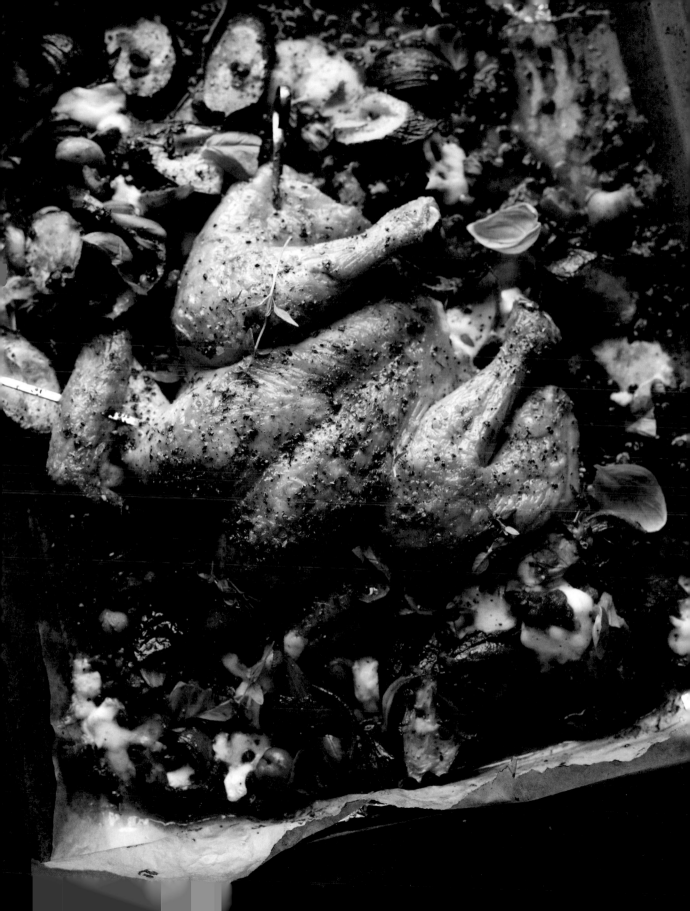

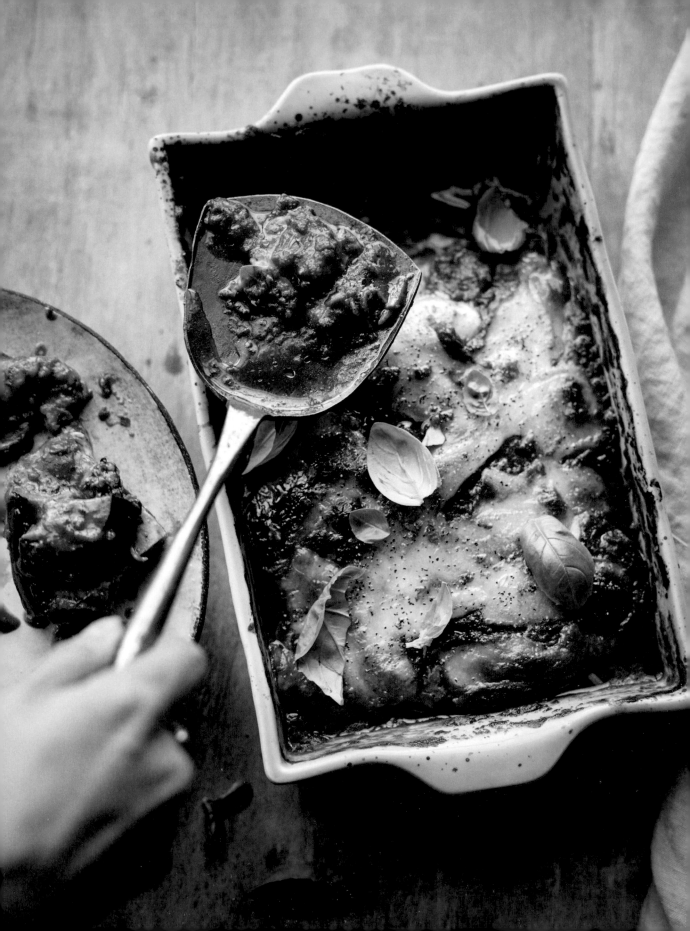

REDUCED-CARB
→GOOD TO FREEZE

CHEAT'S CHICKEN PARMIGIANA

This version is much easier to make than a proper parmigiana and it's low carb so you can pile on the cheese. Serve it with a nice big salad or some steamed greens.

→PREP 15 MINS
→COOK 45 MINS

4 skinless chicken breasts

2 tsp olive oil

salt and pepper

2 medium aubergines, cut lengthways into about 10 slices

600g tinned chopped tomatoes

50g tomato puree

1½ tsp dried oregano

large bunch of basil, plus extra for garnish

1 tbsp balsamic vinegar

300g pizza mozzarella

big salad or steamed greens, to serve

Equipment

30 x 18cm ovenproof baking dish

Preheat your oven to 190°C (fan 170°C/gas mark 5).

Lay a piece of cling film over a chopping board and place two of the chicken breasts on top. Lay a second piece of cling film over the breasts, then use a blunt object – a rolling pin, meat mallet or even your fists – to bash the breasts until they are about half the thickness they were. Repeat the process with the other two breasts.

Heat up a large griddle pan over a medium to high heat. Drizzle the chicken breasts with the olive oil, season with salt and pepper, then carefully lay a couple of breasts at a time onto the hot griddle (if you have a massive griddle then add as many as you can fit in without overcrowding the pan). Sear the chicken for about 1 minute on each side, or until the flesh is nicely browned in places. You are not aiming to cook the breasts through at this point. When the breasts are browned, transfer them to a plate and repeat the process with the remaining chicken breasts.

When you have browned off the chicken, griddle the aubergine slices, again drizzling them with a little olive oil and seasoning with salt and pepper before cooking them in batches. The aubergine slices will need about 2 minutes on each side, until they begin to soften.

When you have a pile of browned chicken and aubergine slices, make the tomato sauce by mixing together the chopped tomatoes, tomato puree, dried oregano, basil, balsamic vinegar and a good pinch of salt and pepper. ➡

CHEAT'S CHICKEN
PARMIGIANA (CONTINUED)

To construct your parmigiana, spread one third of the tomato sauce on the bottom of a baking dish, then lay half of the cooked aubergines on top. Cut the mozzarella into 3mm slices and then lay half of them on top of the aubergine and season with salt and pepper. Place the chicken breasts on the cheese, overlapping them a little.

Lay the remaining aubergine on top of the chicken, pour the rest of the tomato sauce over the top and then lay the rest of the mozzarella on top of the sauce. Cover the dish with tin foil and bake in the preheated oven for 15 minutes. Remove the foil and cook for a further 15 minutes or until the mozzarella has melted and is turning golden.

Garnish your cheesy treat with a few extra basil leaves and serve up with a big bowl of salad or steamed greens.

★ *IF YOU DON'T HAVE A GRIDDLE PAN, HAVE NO FEAR: YOU CAN COOK THE BASHED CHICKEN BREASTS JUST AS WELL USING A NORMAL FRYING PAN.*

Serves 4

REDUCED-CARB

TOAD IN THE HOLE

This is one of my favourite meals as it reminds me of growing up, when I used to stay around my Nan's after school. She always turned up to meet me with a bag of sweets and would make me toad in the hole. It's really easy to make and well worth the wait.

➧ PREP 10 MINS
➧ COOK 40 MINS

3 eggs
275ml semi-skimmed milk
salt
125g plain flour
2½ tbsp sunflower oil
10 sausages
steamed greens, to serve

For the sage and onion gravy
½ tbsp sunflower oil
1 large onion, finely sliced
6 sage leaves, finely sliced
1 tbsp plain flour
splash of sherry vinegar
500ml chicken or beef stock

Equipment
29 x 21cm heavy-based baking dish or 25cm ovenproof skillet

Beat the eggs and the milk together, adding a little salt as you whisk. Tip the flour into a bowl and make a small well in the middle. Pour in the milk-and-egg mixture. Use a whisk to gently combine until you end up with a perfectly smooth batter. Leave to stand while you prepare the rest of the ingredients.

Preheat your oven to 210°C (fan 190°C/gas mark 6). Pour 2 tablespoons of the oil into the baking dish or ovenproof skillet and slide it into the oven to heat up for at least 10 minutes.

Meanwhile, pour ½ tablespoon of the oil into a frying pan over a medium to high heat. Add the sausages and briefly brown them all over – it isn't necessary to cook them through at this point because they will finish cooking in the oven.

By now the oil in the baking dish should be piping hot so carefully remove the dish from the oven and, working quickly and carefully, lay the browned sausages into the dish. Give the batter one last whisk, then pour it over the top of the sausages before quickly sliding the dish back into the oven. Bake the toad in the hole for 35 minutes. ➧

★ *HEATING THE BAKING DISH OR SKILLET BEFORE YOU START COOKING IS THE SECRET TO THE RISE, SO DON'T SKIP THAT STEP!*

TOAD IN THE HOLE (CONTINUED)

Meanwhile, make the onion gravy by heating up ½ tablespoon of oil in a saucepan over a medium heat and adding the sliced onion. Sprinkle in a pinch of salt and cook the onion slowly for about 10 minutes, stirring regularly, until very soft and lightly browned.

Stir in the sage leaves and the flour and, stirring almost constantly, cook for 45 seconds before adding the splash of vinegar, boiling it until it has almost disappeared. Gradually pour in the stock, stirring it well before adding more, to avoid lumps in the gravy. When all the stock is in the pan, bring the gravy to the boil and then keep it warm until you are ready to eat.

After 35 minutes, the toad in the hole should have risen beautifully. Take it straight to the table with the gravy and some steamed greens, and show it off to your mates.

★ *THIS GRAVY IS A TOTAL WINNER – IT WORKS WITH ALMOST ANY MEAT.*

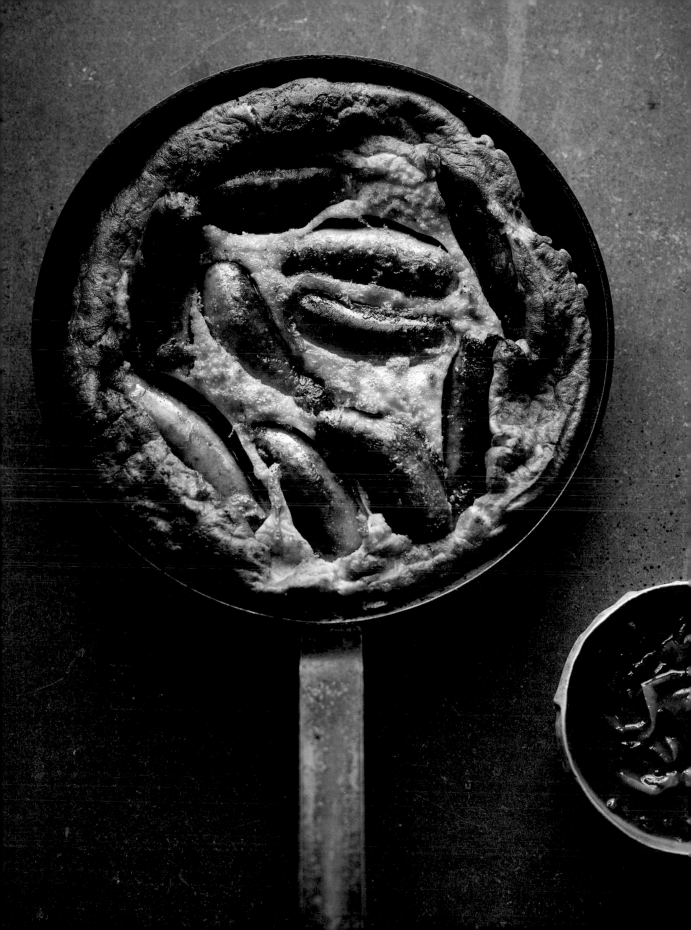

REDUCED-CARB

CHICKEN, SAUSAGE & FENNEL TRAY BAKE

Here's another quick-prep meal that gets thrown into one tray. I love cooking this way because there's less washing up to do!

→**PREP 10 MINS**
→**COOK 1 HR**

1½ tbsp coconut oil
4 chicken thighs, bone-in and skin-on
salt and pepper
12 sausages
1 red onion, cut into 8 wedges
2 fennel bulbs, cut into 8 wedges each
4 cloves garlic, bashed and left whole
2 courgettes, cut into 2cm chunks
4 sprigs of thyme
180g halloumi, cut into 2cm chunks
16 cherry tomatoes, on the vine if possible

To serve
rocket
2 lemons, quartered

Preheat your oven to 190°C (fan 170°C/gas mark 5).

Dollop the coconut oil onto a roasting tray and slide it into the oven to heat for 10 minutes.

Season the chicken thighs all over with salt and pepper. When the coconut oil is hot, carefully slide the tray out of the oven and lay the chicken thighs in, skin-side down. Place the sausages around the thighs. Slide the tray back into the oven and roast the meat for 15 minutes.

Take the tray out of the oven and flip over the sausages, keeping the chicken thighs cooking skin-side down. Scatter over the red onion and fennel wedges, and chuck in the garlic, courgettes, thyme sprigs and chunks of halloumi. Give the mixture a rough stir around, being careful not to turn the thighs. Slide the tray back into the oven and continue to roast for 25 minutes.

Remove the tray from the oven again and give everything a good stir. Flip over the chicken thighs. Plonk the cherry tomatoes on top and slide the tray back into the oven for a final 10-minute blast.

Finally, remove the tray from the oven and this time keep it out. Serve up the chicken and sausages with a big pile of rocket and a good squeeze of lemon.

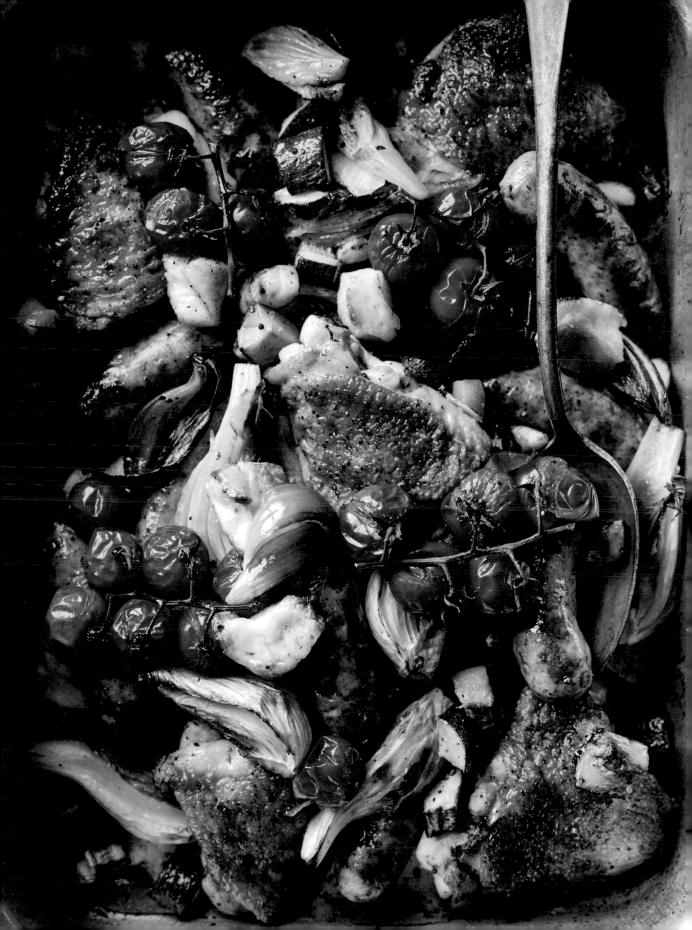

REDUCED-CARB
➡ GOOD TO FREEZE

➡ PREP 15 MINS
➡ COOK 45 MINS

500g lamb mince
250g beef mince
50g breadcrumbs
1 egg
12 pitted black olives, roughly chopped
20g pine nuts, roughly chopped
small bunch of parsley, finely chopped, plus extra for garnish
2 jarred red peppers (about 100g), drained and roughly chopped into small pieces
1 tbsp olive oil
1 red onion, diced
1 x 400g tin of chopped tomatoes
salt and pepper
2 x 110g balls of mozzarella

To serve
mint leaves, roughly chopped
salad or steamed green beans

JOE'S BIG MEATY BALLS

I've combined both beef and lamb mince in this recipe and it works so well. It gives the meatballs so much more flavour. I think once you try these you'll be coming back for more.

Preheat your oven to 180°C (fan 160°C/gas mark 4).

Place the lamb and beef mince into a bowl and add the breadcrumbs. Crack in the egg and chuck in the olives, pine nuts, chopped parsley and red peppers.

Get your hands stuck in and knead all of the ingredients together until the mixture is well combined. With damp hands, shape the mixture into 12 large balls and set aside.

Heat the olive oil in a large ovenproof pan over a medium to high heat. When the oil is hot, chuck in the red onion and fry, stirring regularly for 2 minutes. Tip in the chopped tomatoes along with a quarter tin of water. Season with salt and pepper and bring to the boil.

Place the meatballs in the sauce and simmer for 10 minutes, then carefully flip them over with a large spoon. Tear up the mozzarella balls and lay a little piece on top of each meat ball. Any remaining cheese can be scattered in the sauce.

Slide your pan into the oven and bake for 20 minutes, until the meatballs are fully cooked through and the cheese has melted and turned golden brown on top. Scatter over the mint leaves and remaining chopped parsley and serve with a helping of salad or steamed green beans.

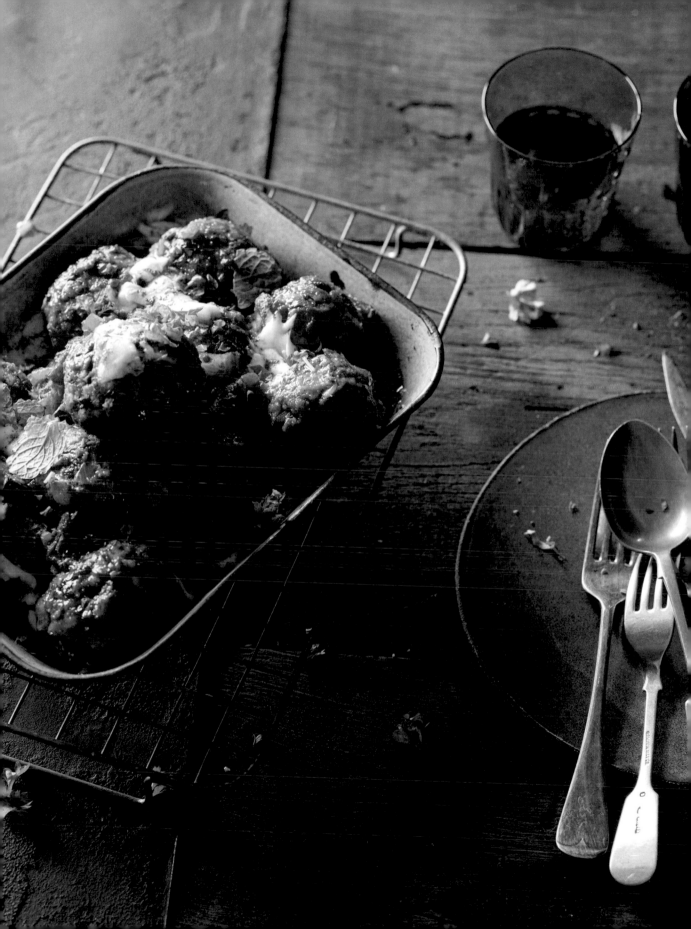

Serves 4

REDUCED-CARB

PORK CHOPS WITH CHEESY CHORIZO SPROUTS

I used to run a mile when I saw brussels sprouts on my plate but now I've realized just how good they are when cooked with other stuff like chorizo and cheese. If you're not a sprout fan, you will be after this.

◆PREP 15 MINS
◆COOK 35 MINS

600g brussels sprouts, cut in half
80g chorizo, cut into 5mm pieces
knob of butter
1 onion, diced
2 cloves garlic, diced
100ml white wine
150ml chicken stock
125ml double cream
65g gruyère, grated
80g cheddar, grated
small bunch of parsley, roughly chopped
salt and pepper
4 pork chops
4 large handfuls of watercress, to serve

Preheat your oven to 190°C (fan 170°C/gas mark 5) and bring a pan of water to the boil over a high heat.

Drop in the sprouts. Bring the water back up to the boil and simmer for 6 minutes, until the sprouts are just tender. Drain them in a sieve or colander and cool under cold running water.

Meanwhile, tip the chorizo into a dry pan over a low to medium heat and fry for about 6 minutes, or until crisp. Transfer the cooked chorizo to a piece of kitchen roll to remove excess oil.

Melt the butter in a second pan over a medium to high heat. When it is hot, add the onion to the pan and cook, stirring regularly for 5 minutes, or until it starts to soften. Add the garlic, and continue to stir-fry for a further 3 minutes, reducing the heat if the ingredients start to burn.

When the onion and garlic have softened, increase the heat to maximum. Pour in the white wine and reduce by half. Pour in the stock and reduce the liquid by about a half again.

Lower the heat to medium and pour in the cream. Bring to the boil and then take the pan off the heat. Stir in the cheese and parsley along with a little salt and pepper.

Tip the cooked sprouts into a baking dish and pour the sauce over the top. Give the sprouts a little jiggle to coat them fully, then scatter over the chorizo and slide the tray into the oven. Bake for 25 minutes, until browning a little on top.

While the sprouts are in the oven, cook your pork chops under the grill for about 8 minutes on each side, or until they are fully cooked through. Turn off the grill, shut the door and leave to rest in the warm oven until you're ready to eat.

When the sprouts are ready, slide them out and serve with the pork chops and handfuls of watercress.

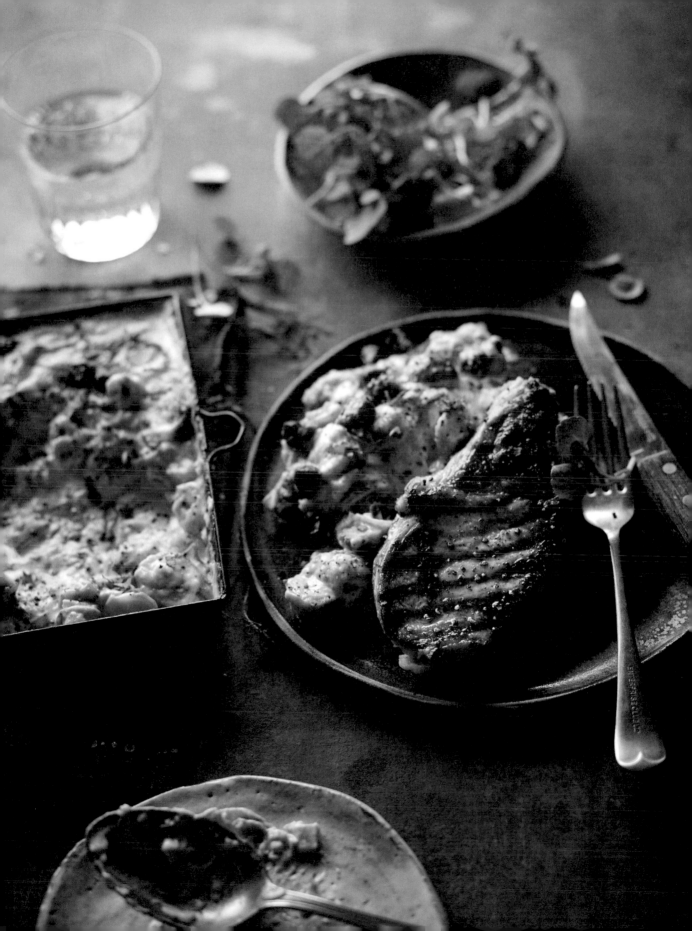

**REDUCED-CARB
→LOW & SLOW**

PULLED PORK
WITH FENNEL SALAD

I know this takes ages to make but truly melt-in-the-mouth pulled pork requires patience. You'll be amazed at how good this tastes, so invite some friends over and give this a go.

**→PREP 10 MINS
→COOK 4 HRS 30 MINS**

1½ tbsp olive oil

1 tsp sweet smoked paprika

1 tsp ground cumin

salt and pepper

1.75kg piece of rolled pork shoulder

2 red onions

4 sprigs of thyme

juice of ½ orange

2 bulbs of fennel, finely sliced

1 carrot, cut into matchsticks

¼ red cabbage, finely sliced

2½ tbsp mayonnaise

2 tsp white wine vinegar

½ tsp caraway seeds

40g walnuts, roughly chopped

Preheat your oven to 200°C (fan 180°C/gas mark 6).

Mix together the oil, paprika and cumin in a bowl along with a generous pinch of salt and pepper. Rub the mixture all over the pork, then place it into a roasting tray. Slide it into your oven and roast for 20 minutes.

Remove the joint from the oven and reduce the temperature to 160°C (fan 140°C/gas mark 3). Roll out a large piece of tin foil and lay a piece of baking parchment on top of that. Roughly slice one of the red onions and place it in the middle of the paper. Drop the thyme sprigs on top. Using two forks, pick up the pork and place it on top of the onion and thyme, then move the whole lot back into the roasting tray.

Draw the sides of the parchment up around the pork, then squeeze over the orange juice. Seal the tin foil together and return the pork to the oven to cook for 4 hours.

When the pork has 20 minutes to go, prepare your fennel salad. Finely slice the second red onion and slide it into a large bowl with the other prepped vegetables. Add the mayonnaise, white wine vinegar, caraway seeds and walnuts, and stir until well combined. Set aside until you're ready to eat.

When the pork is ready, remove it from the oven and leave it to sit for 10 minutes. Rip open the tin foil and transfer to a big serving dish. Use two forks to pull the pork apart, then serve with the salad and get stuck in.

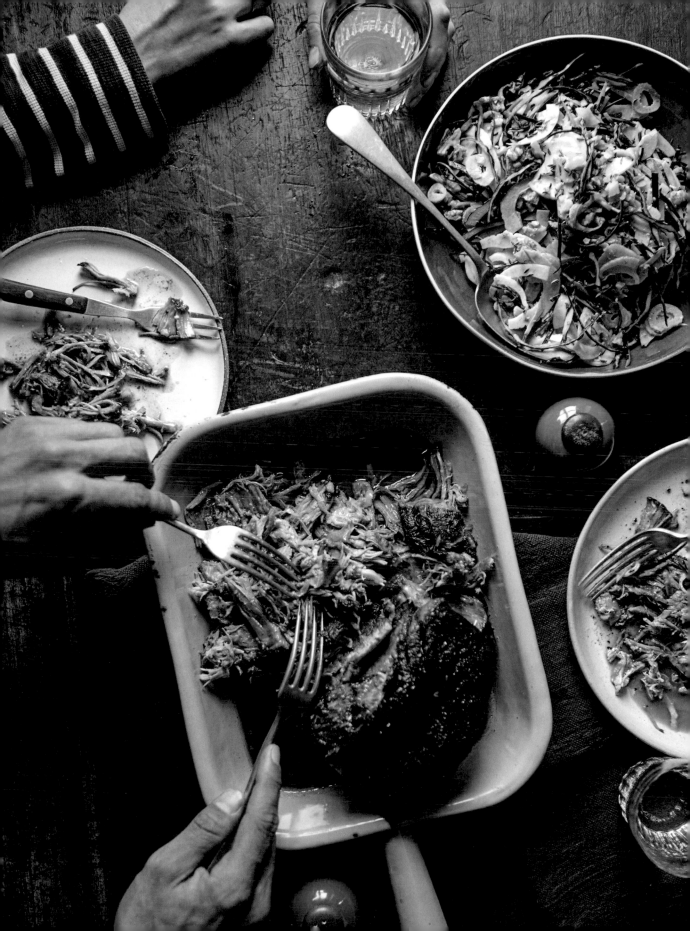

REDUCED-CARB
➤**LOW & SLOW**
➤**GOOD TO FREEZE**

➤**PREP 12 MINS**
➤**COOK 2 HRS 40 MINS**

1 tbsp olive oil

2 leeks, cut into chunks

2 large carrots, cut into long sticks

2 parsnips, cut into long sticks

2 red onions, cut into large wedges

6 cloves garlic, unpeeled and bashed

1 x 400g tin of chopped tomatoes

3 sprigs of rosemary

1 leg of lamb (around 1.9kg)

salt and pepper

bacon greens (see page 97), to serve

Equipment
hob-proof roasting tin

LAMB LEG POT ROAST

This is perfect for a Sunday roast as it's really easy to make and can feed a small army. It all goes in one big tray so once the prep is done you can relax and enjoy.

Preheat your oven to 170°C (fan 150°C/gas mark 3).

Place the hob-proof roasting tin over a medium heat and pour in the oil. Add the leeks, carrots, parsnips, red onions and garlic and fry, stirring regularly for 5 minutes.

Pour the chopped tomatoes and 100ml of water into the tin and bring to the boil. Lay the rosemary sprigs in the middle of the tomato mixture and then place the lamb leg on top. Season the lamb with a decent amount of salt and pepper.

Cover your tin tightly with tin foil and slide it into the oven to cook for 2 hours 30 minutes, or until the leg is lovely and tender.

Serve with bacon greens for meal that will satisfy everybody's tastebuds.

★ *IF YOU DON'T HAVE A HOB-PROOF ROASTING TRAY THEN START THE VEG IN A SAUCEPAN AND TRANSFER TO A ROASTING TRAY. IT MIGHT TAKE AN EXTRA 10–15 MINUTES IN THE OVEN.*

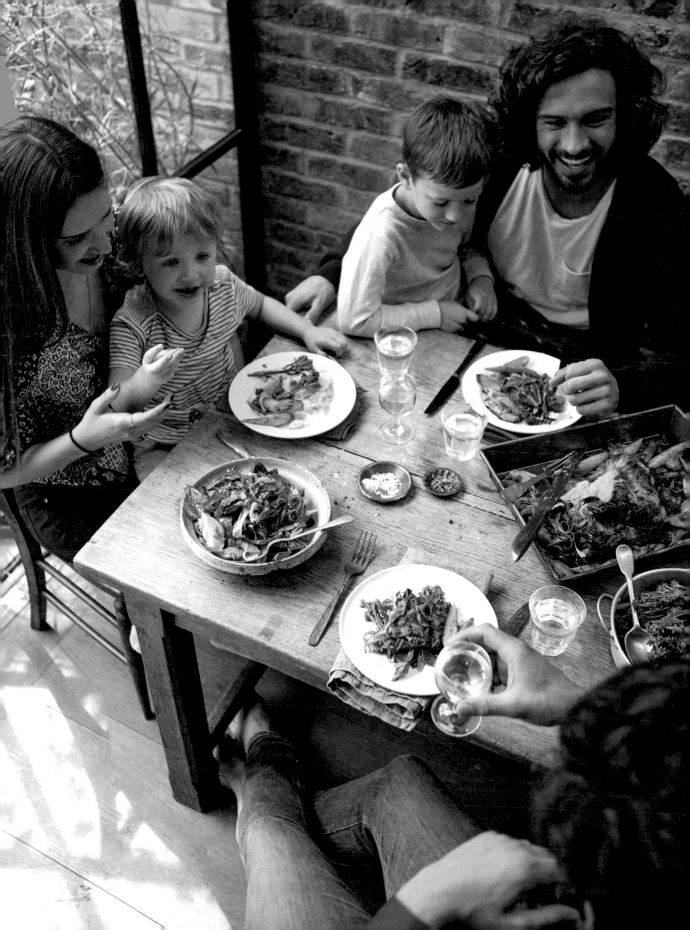

REDUCED-CARB
➡**GOOD TO FREEZE**

COQ AU STOCK

This is my lean version of Coq au vin, without the wine. It's easy to make and makes you look like a good cook so friends will be well impressed. If you don't have one massive frying pan, you can just split the recipe between two smaller pans.

➡**PREP 10 MINS**
➡**COOK 40 MINS**

knob of butter
1 tbsp olive oil
6 chicken leg portions, bone-in and skin-on
1 onion, diced
6 rashers of streaky bacon, cut into 1cm slices
4 cloves garlic, bashed and left whole
200g mushrooms, roughly chopped
salt and pepper
250ml chicken stock
175g green beans, trimmed
100g crème fraiche

To serve
½ bunch of chives, finely chopped
½ bunch of parsley, roughly chopped

Melt the butter and oil in a very large frying pan over a medium to high heat. When the butter is bubbling, lay the chicken portions into the pan to brown, skin-side down. Aim for a deep golden brown all over – this should take about 8 minutes.

When the legs are brown, transfer them onto a plate. The chicken will have rendered fat and juice, so carefully tip a little of the liquid out of the pan and discard. Scrape the chopped onion and bacon slices into the pan and fry over a medium to high heat for about 4 minutes, or until the onion starts to soften.

Add the garlic and mushrooms along with a pinch of salt and pepper and continue stir-frying for a further 2 minutes.

Lay the chicken pieces back into the pan, skin-side down, and pour in the chicken stock. Crank up the heat and bring the liquid to the boil, then lower the heat to a simmer. Place a lid on top and leave the chicken to cook for 25 minutes.

After 20 minutes, carefully remove the lid and scatter the green beans over the top, then place the lid back on and cook for a further 5 minutes, until the chicken is fully cooked. Check by slicing into one of the larger pieces to make sure the meat is white all the way through, with no raw pink bits left.

Stir in the crème fraiche and bring the sauce to the boil one last time. Scatter with the chopped chives and parsley and serve.

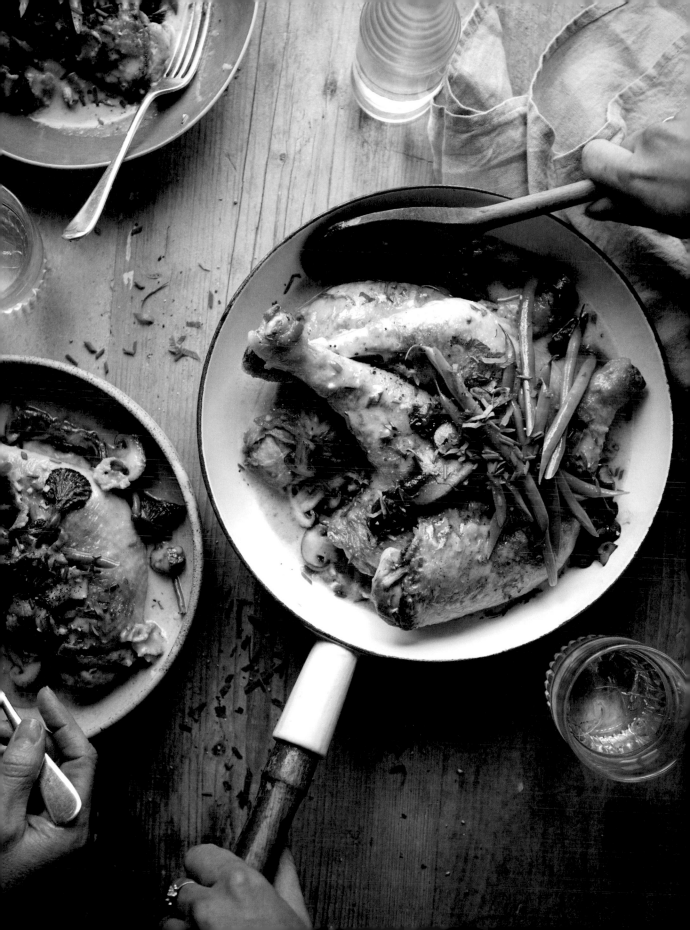

REDUCED-CARB
→ MAKE AHEAD

→ PREP 15 MINS
→ COOK 1 HR

½ tbsp coconut oil

2 red onions, diced

2 celery sticks, diced

3 cloves garlic, finely chopped

2 red chillies, de-seeded and finely chopped

500g reduced-fat lamb mince

1 tsp ground cinnamon

1½ tsp dried oregano

1 tbsp tomato puree

1 x 400g tin chopped tomatoes

salt and pepper

4 peppers (any combo of red, orange and yellow ones)

a little olive oil, for drizzling

180g pizza mozzarella, cut into 8 slices

large salad, to serve

SPICY LAMB-STUFFED PEPPERS

These really do taste as good as they look. If you have any leftovers, stick them in a box and you can reheat them the next day in the microwave for lunch.

Preheat your oven to 190°C (fan 170°C/gas mark 5).

Melt the coconut oil in a large saucepan over a medium to high heat. When it is hot, add the onions, celery, garlic and chillies and cook, stirring regularly for 5 minutes.

Meanwhile, warm another frying pan over a maximum heat for 2–3 minutes. When it is smoking hot, carefully lay the lamb mince into the pan and fry hard, without stirring. After 1 minute, turn the meat carefully. The lamb will release juices and oil and will cease to brown – at this point get stuck in with a wooden spoon and break up the meat.

When the onions have softened in the saucepan, add the cinnamon, oregano, and tomato puree and stir. Tip the browned mince straight into the saucepan and stir until well mixed.

Pour in the chopped tomatoes, season with a good amount of salt and pepper, then clamp on the lid and leave to cook, covered, for 10 minutes. Give it a stir every now and then and reduce the heat a little if you think it may be burning.

While the lamb is cooking, cut each pepper in half through its stalk and carefully remove as much of the white inner skin and seeds as possible. Lay the pepper halves, cut-side up, on a baking tray, drizzle with olive oil and roast in the oven for 15 minutes, until starting to soften, but still holding their shape.

When the lamb has been simmering for 10 minutes, remove the lid and simmer for 2 minutes. Take the pan off the heat and divide the lamb mince mixture between the pepper halves.

Top each filled pepper half with a thick slice of mozzarella, then slide the tray back into the oven and bake for 25 minutes, until the cheese is golden and oozing. Serve with a generous salad.

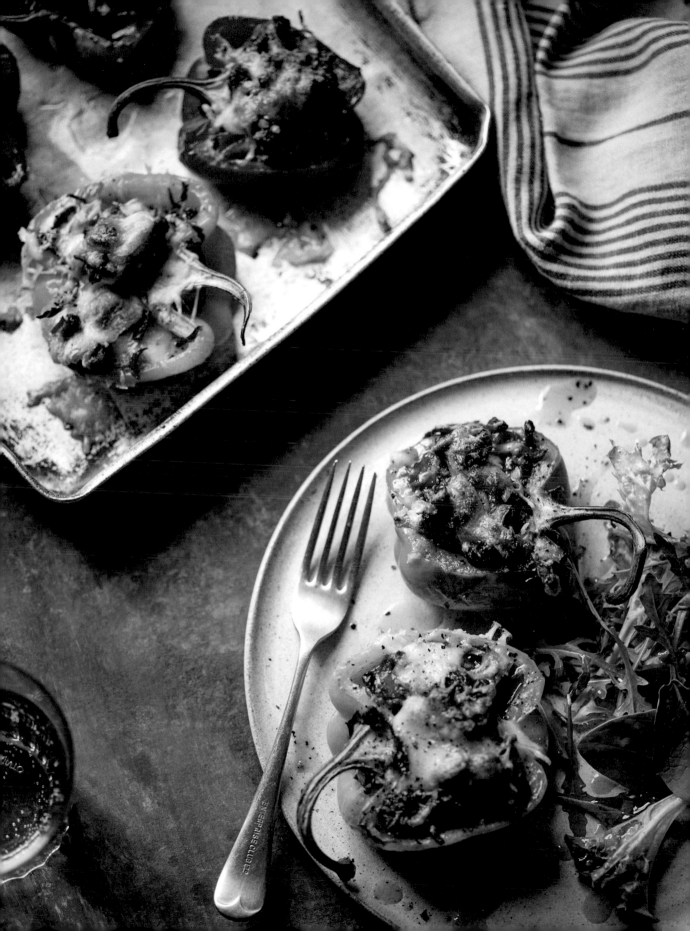

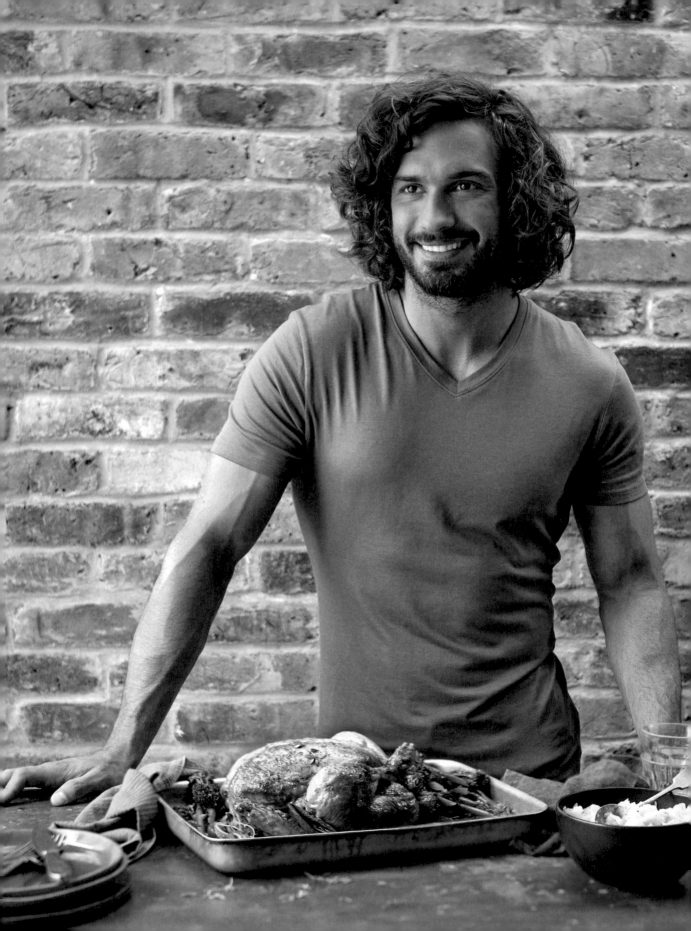

REDUCED-CARB
→LOW & SLOW

→PREP 20 MINS
→COOK 1 HR 30 MINS

1 good-quality whole chicken
(around 1.5kg)
4 sprigs of thyme
5 stalks of sage
1 onion, cut into wedges
juice of 1 lemon
1 litre chicken stock
2 celeriac, peeled and roughly
cubed
40g butter
salt and pepper
1 tbsp cornflour

For the bacon greens
10g butter
3 rashers of smoked streaky
bacon, cut into 1cm strips
2 spring greens, tough stalks
removed, leaves roughly
shredded
220g midget trees (tender-stem
broccoli), cut in half, stalk and all

ROAST CHICKEN, MASH
& BACON GREENS

If you want a healthier version of a Sunday roast, then
look no further. I've used celeriac instead of potato to
make a low-carb mash and added some more flavour to
the greens by frying them with bacon.

Preheat your oven to 180°C (fan 160°C/gas mark 4).

Place the chicken into a roasting tin and place three of the
thyme sprigs and four of the sage stalks into its cavity with the
onion wedges. Squeeze the lemon juice over the chicken and
pour 500ml of the stock into the tin.

Slide the prepped chicken into the oven and roast for about
1 hour 10 minutes, or until the chicken is cooked through –
check by slicing into the thickest part of the thigh to make
sure that the juices run clear. When the chicken is cooked,
transfer it onto a plate and cover with tin foil to rest for
around 15 minutes.

While the chicken is roasting, bring a large pan of water to the
boil. Add the celeriac cubes and simmer for about 15 minutes,
or until the pieces are very tender. Drain the celeriac in a sieve
or colander and leave to steam dry.

Add 40g of the butter to the same saucepan and allow it to melt
in the residual heat. Give the celeriac one more shake and then
tip it into the pan with the butter. Season with a good pinch of
salt and pepper and then mash. Don't mash up the celeriac too
much – it is nice to retain some texture. Keep warm until ready
to serve. ➡

ROAST CHICKEN, MASH & BACON GREENS (CONTINUED)

About 15 minutes before the chicken is ready, make the bacon greens by melting 10g butter in a large saucepan. When it is hot, add the bacon and fry over a medium to high heat for 2 minutes.

Add the spring greens and midget trees along with a splash of water and put a lid on top. Steam the greens for 5 minutes, or until just tender. Keep warm until ready to serve.

While the chicken is resting, pour the liquid from the roasting tin into a measuring jug and make it up to 500ml with the remaining chicken stock. Put the roasting tin or a saucepan onto the hob and pour the liquid in.

Mix the cornflour with about 2 tablespoons of water or stock and pour it into the warming mixture in the tin or saucepan (do not add the cornflour if the mixture is boiling, otherwise it will go lumpy) and then increase the heat, stirring constantly until your gravy has thickened.

Strip the leaves from the remaining thyme and sage stalks, finely chop them up and add them to the gravy. Serve up and enjoy.

Serves 4-6

REDUCED-CARB
➡ BBQ

STICKY BBQ RIBS WITH DIRTY CORN

These ribs are off-the-scale crazy tasty. Pull this recipe out at your next barbecue if you want to impress your mates. I think the secret is the Worcestershire sauce.

➡ PREP 15 MINS,
 PLUS MARINATING TIME
➡ COOK 30 MINS

1 tbsp coconut oil
1 large red onion, diced
3cm fresh ginger, diced
2 tbsp molasses
225ml Worcestershire sauce
75g tomato puree
1.5kg spare ribs
4 corn on the cobs
3 tbsp mayonnaise
40g parmesan, grated
½ bunch of chives, finely sliced
cayenne or paprika, for dusting

Equipment
food processor

Melt the oil in a saucepan over a medium to high heat. When it is hot, add the red onion and ginger and cook for about 5 minutes, or until the onion is soft.

Pour in the molasses, Worcestershire sauce, tomato puree and 75ml of water and bring to the boil. Reduce the heat to a simmer and cook for 5 more minutes. Leave to cool a little and then blitz in a food processor until you reach a smooth sauce. Pour the barbecue sauce over the ribs and leave to marinate for at least 2 hours.

Bring a saucepan of water to the boil and simmer the corn on the cobs for 6 minutes, or until the kernels start to feel tender. Drain thoroughly.

Fire up the barbecue, if using. When you are ready to eat, cook the ribs over a medium to hot barbecue for about 6 minutes on each side, putting a lid on if you have one. If you're using a griddle pan, cook the ribs for about 6 minutes on each side.

Check the ribs are cooked through by cutting into the flesh near the tip of the bone to make sure there are no raw pink bits left. If you're unsure, transfer them to the oven, preheated to 220°C (fan 200°C/gas mark 7), for another 5 minutes.

When the ribs are cooked, remove them to a plate and leave to rest until you're ready to eat.

Meanwhile, brown the corn on the barbecue or on a hot griddle pan for about 5 minutes. As soon as the corn is ready, spread over a little mayonnaise, sprinkle with parmesan and chives, and finish with a dusting of cayenne or paprika.

Serve up the ribs with the dirty corn and dive in.

SEE PHOTOS OVERLEAF ➡

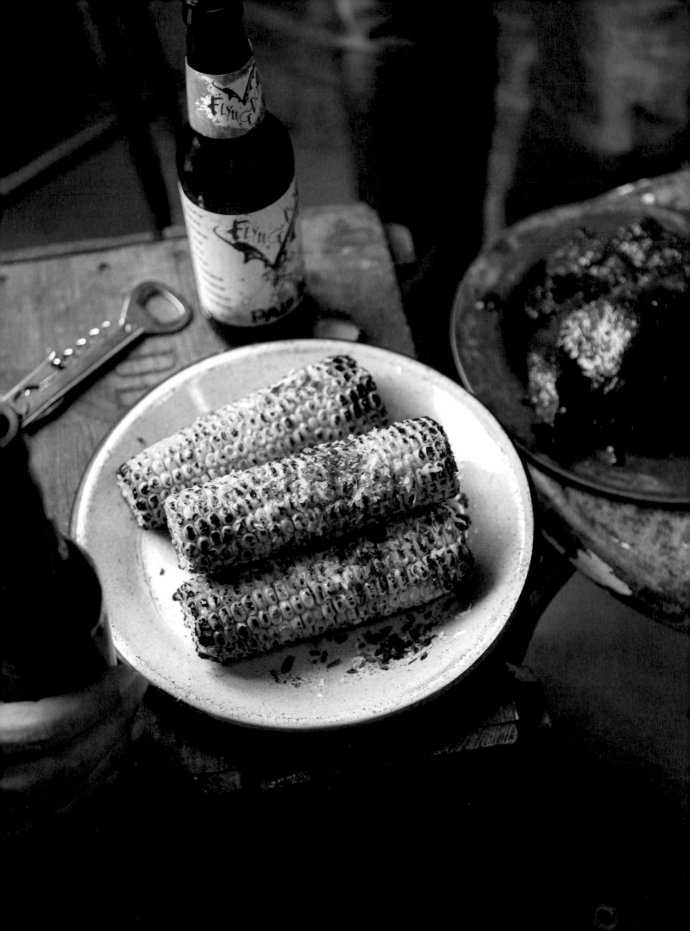

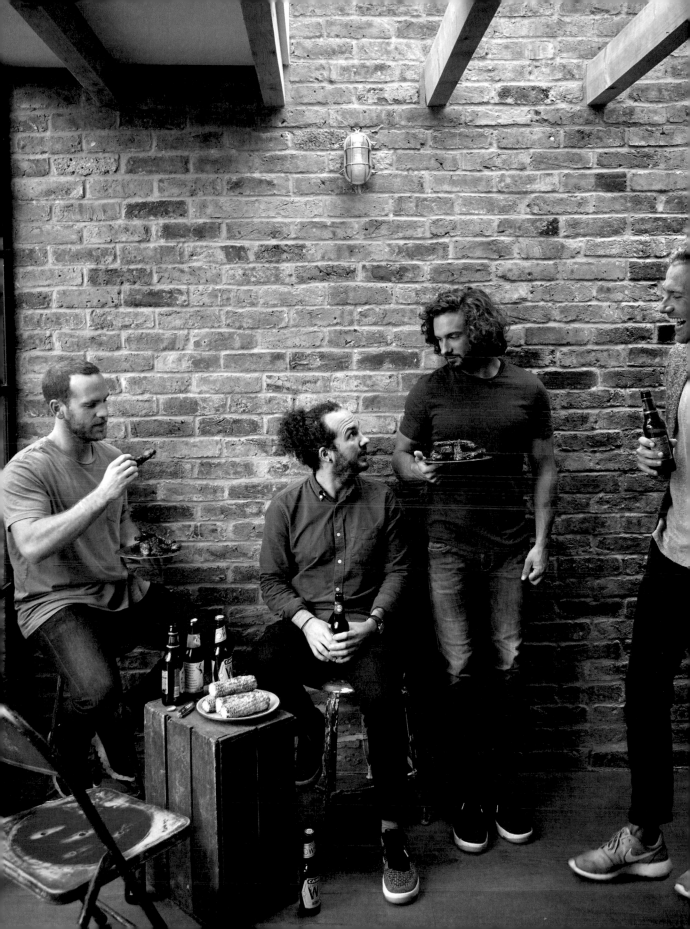

REDUCED-CARB
→ BBQ

LAMB WITH BLACK OLIVES & ROSEMARY

If you don't often cook with lamb, maybe give this recipe a go. It makes a nice change to eating chicken or beef and you'll be surprised how good it tastes.

→ PREP 10 MINS
→ COOK 10 MINS

salt and pepper
4 x 125g lamb leg steaks
12 pitted black olives, roughly cut in half
10 cherry tomatoes, sliced in half
2 sprigs of rosemary, needles only, finely chopped
1 red chilli, de-seeded and finely sliced
½ small bunch of basil, roughly chopped
1½ tbsp pine nuts
2 tbsp olive oil
3 spring onions, finely sliced
green salad, to serve

Fire up your barbecue or preheat your griddle pan to a high heat. Season the steaks and lay them onto the preheated barbecue or griddle pan. Cook for 3 minutes on each side.

While the lamb is cooking, mix together the remaining ingredients in a large bowl to create a dressing.

As soon as the steaks have had their cooking time, transfer them straight into the bowl with the dressing, cover with tin foil and leave to rest for 15 minutes.

Divide the rested steaks between four plates, toss together the ingredients in the bowl with the resting juices, then pile the dressing high on top of the steaks.

Serve up with a nice big green salad.

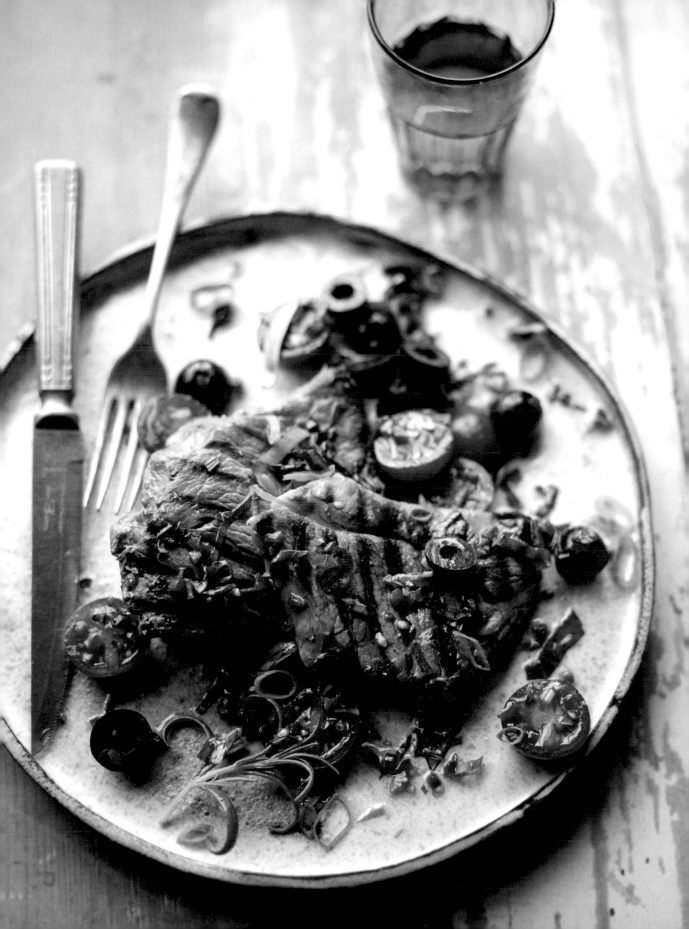

REDUCED-CARB
⮞BBQ

SPATCHCOCK CHICKEN WITH SPECIAL SAUCE

It may seem a bit daunting to spatchcock your own whole chicken but it's actually really easy and makes it much quicker to cook on the barbecue.

⮞PREP 15 MINS
⮞COOK 25 MINS

1 whole chicken (around 1.5kg)
3 sprigs of rosemary
3 sprigs of thyme
1 x 250g tub of cream cheese
large bunch of basil, leaves only
large bunch of mint, leaves only
large bunch of chives, roughly chopped
1 clove garlic, roughly chopped
salt and pepper
2 avocados, de-stoned and cut into wedges
2 large handfuls of crunchy green salad, roughly chopped
juice of 1 lemon
3 tbsp olive oil

Equipment
food processor

Fire up the barbecue or preheat your oven to 190°C (fan 170°C/gas mark 5).

To spatchcock your chicken, turn it upside down. Using a clean and sharp pair of scissors, cut either side of the backbone and then completely remove it. Turn the chicken over and then put your hands on top. Lean on the chicken to squash it down – at this point it will probably make a bone-cracking noise, but that's okay.

Use a sharp knife to slash the flesh where the breast meets the wing and the thickest part of the thighs – this just helps the chicken to cook evenly.

Lay the chicken skin-side down onto the medium to hot barbecue and grill for about 25 minutes, flipping halfway through. If your barbecue has a lid, then cook the chicken with the lid on. If you're cooking in the oven, place the chicken on a roasting tin and cook for 30 minutes, flipping halfway through. Check that it is cooked by slicing into a thick part of the thigh to make sure the juices run clear.

When the chicken is cooked, transfer it to a large piece of tin foil. Scatter the rosemary and thyme all over the top and wrap the chicken up to rest for 10 minutes.

While the chicken is resting, make the sauce by blitzing the cream cheese, basil, mint, chives and garlic in the food processor until fairly smooth. You may need to add a couple of tablespoons of water to loosen the mixture. Add a good pinch of salt and pepper and tip the sauce into a bowl.

Mix together the avocado wedges and chopped salad, and drizzle with lemon juice and olive oil. Serve your chicken with the avocado salad and delicious sauce.

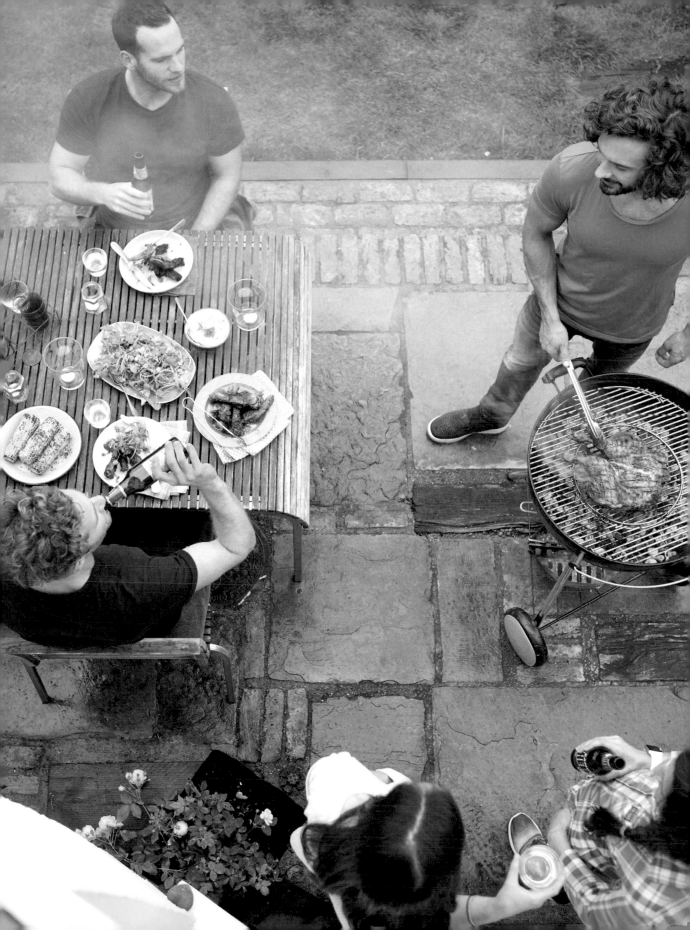

Post Workout

Don't fear the carbs! These recipes are designed to refuel your body after you exercise. They are lower in fat but high in carbohydrate and protein. This is just what your muscles need to rebuild and repair after working out.

Let these whopping great big carb meals be your motivation to smash your workout today. After a HIIT session, there's no greater reward than a Banging breakfast burrito (see page 118) or Phat fish finger sandwich (see page 128). ★

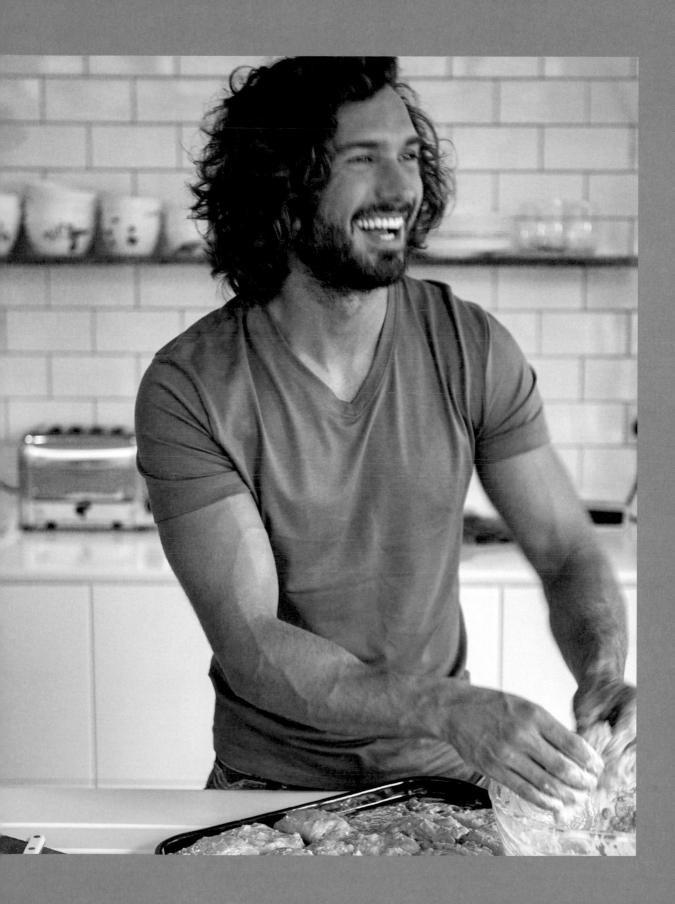

POST-WORKOUT

FRUITY FRENCH TOAST

If you've got a sweet tooth and want a treat after a workout, this is perfect for you. I mean look at the photo. How can you not want to make this one?

◆**PREP 8 MINS**
◆**COOK 20 MINS**

250g strawberries, hulled and cut in half

2–3 tbsp honey

2 eggs

30ml almond milk

¼ tsp mixed spice

1 teaspoon vanilla extract

1 banana, peeled and roughly chopped

1½ tbsp coconut oil

6 slices of thick-cut bread

zero-fat Greek yoghurt, to serve – optional

Equipment
blender

To make the compote, place the strawberries and the honey into a small saucepan over a medium to high heat. Bring to the boil to release a lot of the juices from the strawberries. Simmer for 1 minute before turning the heat off and leaving to cool until ready to serve.

To make the eggy bread, crack the eggs into a blender and add the almond milk, mixed spice, vanilla extract and chopped banana. Blitz until smooth, then tip the mixture into a large bowl.

Unless you have a truly huge frying pan, aim to cook only one eggy bread at a time. Melt a little of the oil in a frying pan over a medium to high heat. Dip one of the slices of bread in the eggy mixture and let it soak for a few seconds, then flip it over and leave it for a few more seconds to absorb.

When the coconut oil is hot, gently lay the soaked slice into the pan and fry for about 2–3 minutes on each side until it turns a dark golden brown. Transfer the cooked eggy bread to a clean piece of kitchen roll to remove the excess oil.

Repeat the process with the remaining oil and slices of bread and then serve with a generous spoonful of the compote and yoghurt, if you fancy it.

★ *ADJUST THE AMOUNT OF HONEY IN THE COMPOTE ACCORDING TO YOUR TASTE AND THE RIPENESS AND SWEETNESS OF THE BERRIES.*

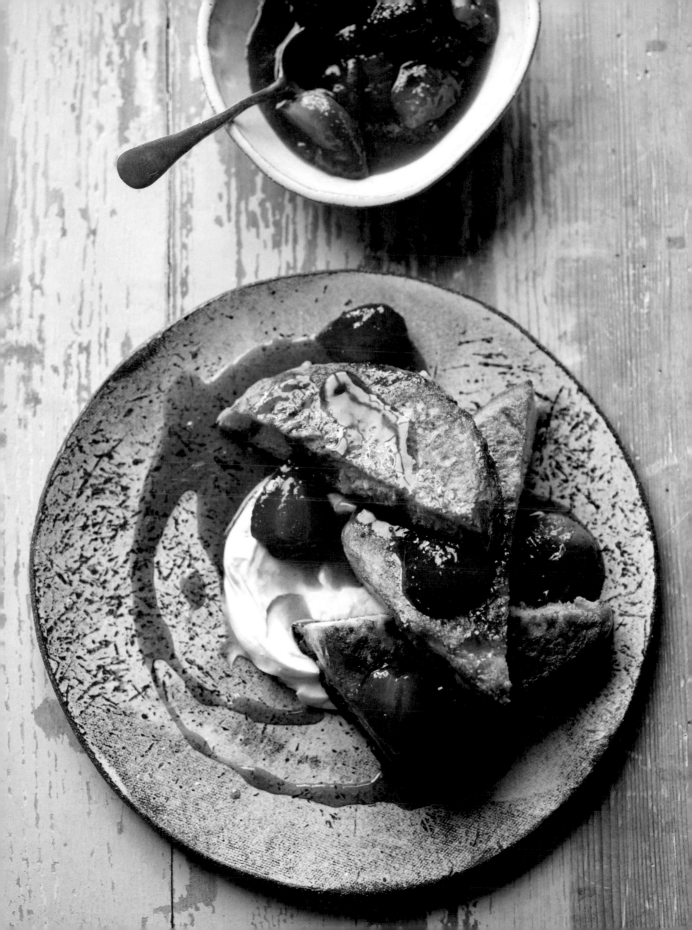

POST-WORKOUT

APPLE & ALMOND POWER PORRIDGE

This porridge is simple, delicious and filling. I find cooking apples have the most flavour but feel free to use your favourite apples.

➧PREP 10 MINS
➧COOK 20 MINS

2 cooking apples, peeled, cored and roughly chopped (about 250g)

130g pitted dates, roughly chopped, plus a few extra to garnish

220g porridge oats

1 tsp ground cinnamon

½ tsp mixed spice

40g vanilla protein powder

920ml almond milk

To serve

a few pecans, roughly chopped

2 tbsp pumpkin seeds

4 tbsp apple compote – optional

Add the chopped apples, dates and a splash of water to a large saucepan over a medium heat. Bring to the boil and then clamp a lid on top and leave the apples to cook for 3 minutes, until totally soft.

Add the oats, cinnamon, mixed spice, protein powder and 850ml of the almond milk and bring gently to the boil. Reduce the heat to a low simmer and cook the porridge for about 15 minutes, or until it is thick and fully cooked through. Add a little more milk along the way if you prefer a runnier texture.

Serve up the steaming porridge and top it with the pecans, pumpkin seeds, a few more chopped dates and some apple compote, if you fancy it.

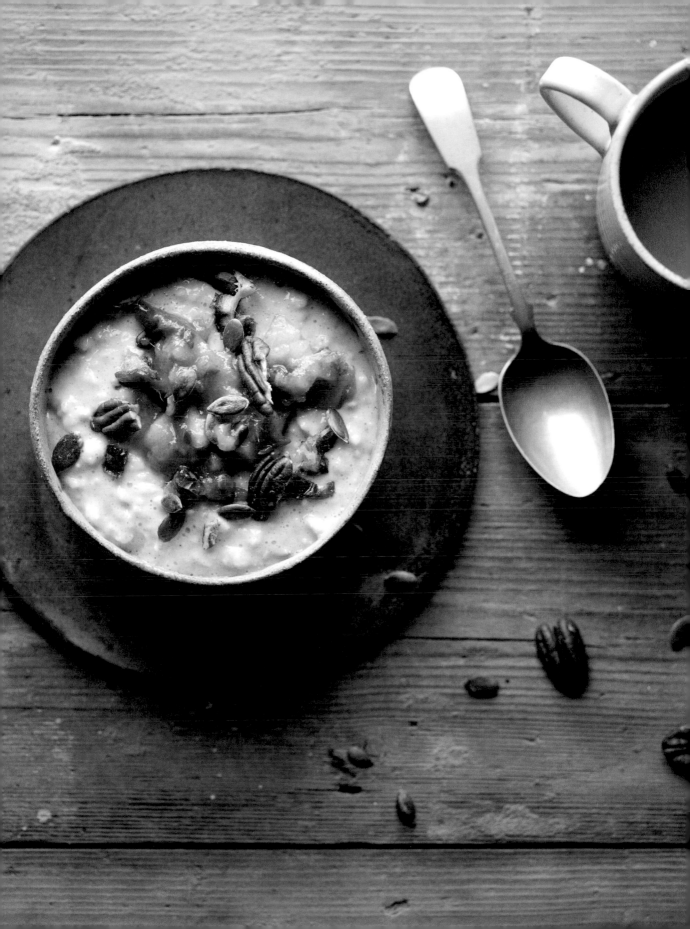

Serves 4

POST-WORKOUT

QUINOA SUPER PORRIDGE

This one will easily keep you going until lunch time. The oat milk tastes lovely but you can use normal milk if you prefer.

➤PREP 5 MINS
➤COOK 30 MINS

175g pitted dates, roughly chopped into small pieces
90g quinoa
90g porridge oats
1 litre oat milk
sliced apple and raspberries, to serve

Chuck the dates into a large saucepan and add about 50ml of water. Place the lid on top and bring to the boil. Simmer with the lid on for 3 minutes, or until the dates are beginning to break up.

Add the quinoa, oats and milk and slowly bring to the boil, stirring regularly. Cook the porridge over a very low heat for 30 minutes, or until the quinoa is cooked.

Serve up the porridge topped with sliced apple and raspberries.

★ *THIS PORRIDGE COULD HAPPILY ABSORB 35–50G OF VANILLA PROTEIN POWDER IF YOU NEED SOME EXTRA FUEL.*

BREAKFAST FRIED RICE

Imagine a bowl with fried rice, sausages, bacon and spring onions. Then imagine adding soy sauce and sesame oil and sticking a fried egg on top of it. Mmm, yes please!

◆PREP 10 MINS
◆COOK 10 MINS

½ tbsp coconut oil

4 chicken sausages, cut into 2cm chunks

2 rashers of back bacon, cut into 1cm slices

4 spring onions, trimmed and finely sliced

4 large mushrooms, roughly chopped into 2cm chunks

½ x 400g tin of butter beans (roughly 250g), drained and rinsed

250g pre-cooked rice

large handful of baby spinach

1½ tbsp light soy sauce

1 tsp sesame oil

2 eggs

3 tbsp tomato ketchup

3 tsp tabasco sauce

Melt half of the oil in a large frying pan over a medium to high heat. When it is hot, chuck in the chicken sausages, bacon, spring onions and mushrooms and fry for 5 minutes. Stir occasionally but allow the ingredients to colour a little bit.

Add the butter beans and the rice to the pan, breaking up the rice with your fingers as you drop it in. Pour in about 2 tablespoons of water and allow it to bubble and heat the rice and beans. Drop in the spinach and continue to stir-fry for about 2 minutes, or until you are sure the meat is cooked through and the rice is hot.

Take the pan off the heat and stir through the soy sauce and sesame oil.

In a second non-stick frying pan, melt the remaining coconut oil over a high heat. When it is hot, crack in the eggs and fry them.

Mix together the ketchup and the tabasco sauce.

Serve up the fried rice on two plates, top with a fried egg each and drizzle over the hot sauce.

Makes 8

AMERICAN-STYLE BLUEBERRY PANCAKES

Everyone on my Instagram goes crazy when I post a stack of protein pancakes, so it only seemed right to include a new pancake recipe. This one will not disappoint. They are so satisfying after a workout and also great as a sweet treat every now and then.

▶PREP 10 MINS
▶COOK 20 MINS

300g plain flour
35g vanilla protein powder
2 tsp baking powder
1 tbsp caster sugar
350ml milk
2 eggs
1–2 tbsp coconut oil, for cooking
400g blueberries, plus extra for scattering

To serve
zero-fat Greek yoghurt
maple syrup

Tip the flour into a bowl and add the protein powder, baking powder and sugar.

Measure out the milk, then crack the eggs straight into the measuring jug. Give the two ingredients a good whisk until well combined. Gradually pour the wet mixture into the dry mixture, stirring or whisking as you go to avoid lumps.

When all the liquid has been incorporated, give the mixture a final whisk until smooth.

Melt a little coconut oil in a good non-stick frying pan over a medium to high heat. When it is hot, pour in one ladleful of the batter, which will spread out across the base of the pan to about 15cm wide and 1–1.5cm thick. Fry the pancake on the first side for 3 minutes, reducing the temperature a little if the pancake starts to burn.

While the pancake is cooking, scatter about an eighth of the blueberries in a single layer over the uncooked surface of the pancake. They will be held in place by the raw batter.

Flip the pancake and cook for a further 2–3 minutes, again upping or reducing the heat as necessary – these pancakes are like most other pancakes in that the first one is often not the best. Remove the pancake to a plate and keep it warm while you repeat the process with the remaining batter and blueberries.

Serve up stacks of your pancakes with a few extra blueberries, Greek yoghurt and a cheeky drizzle of maple syrup.

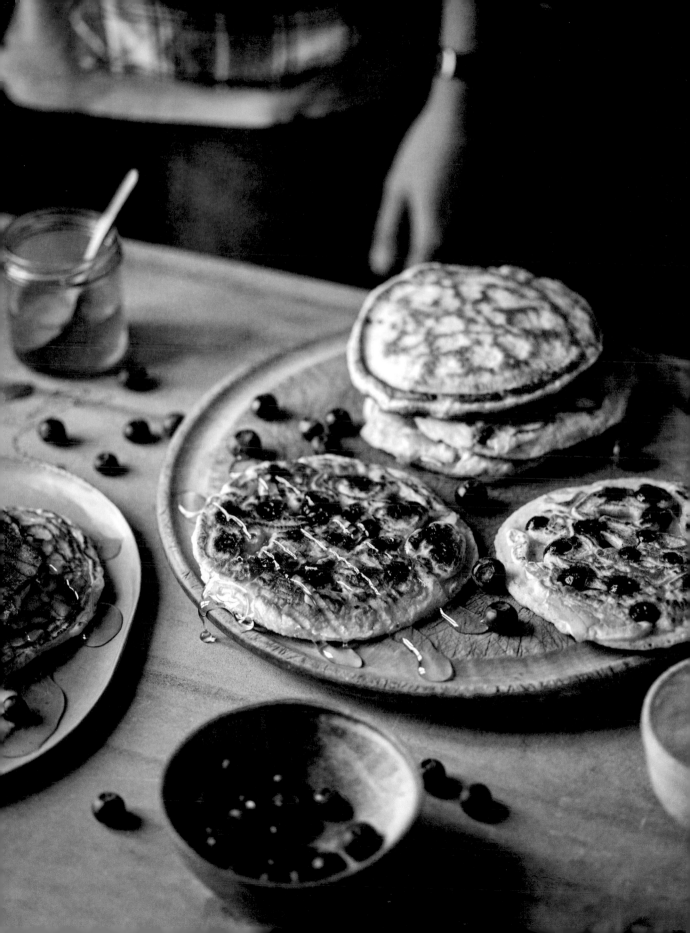

POST-WORKOUT

STICKY COCONUT RICE CAKES

If you like something a little sweet at breakfast then you will love this recipe. There's a bit of prepping and waiting around to begin with but they are well worth the wait.

→ **PREP 12 MINS,
   PLUS COOLING TIME**
→ **COOK 30 MINS**

400g sticky Thai rice
600ml coconut water
4 cardamom pods, bashed
25g soft, light brown sugar
70g vanilla protein powder
2 mangoes, cut into chunks
or wedges
small bunch of mint, leaves only,
finely sliced
1 tbsp coconut oil
maple syrup, to serve – optional

Equipment
30 x 15cm baking tin

Tip the rice into a saucepan, pour over the coconut water, add the cardamom pods and bring to the boil, stirring three or four times. Let the rice boil for 2 minutes, then cover and reduce the heat to its lowest setting. Cook for 20 minutes and then turn off the heat.

Line the baking tin with baking parchment. While the rice is still warm, stir in the sugar and protein powder, making sure they are thoroughly combined. Tip the mixture into the baking tin, use the back of a wet spoon to flatten the surface, and then leave the rice to cool completely.

While the rice is cooling, place the chopped mango into a bowl with the mint. Leave to one side.

When the rice has fully cooled, it will have stuck together in a big, sticky cake. Flip the tray over onto a chopping board in one swift movement and the rice should come out in one piece. Peel off the parchment and cut the rice block up into twelve roughly even pieces.

Melt half of the oil in a large non-stick frying pan over a medium to high heat. When it is hot, carefully lay six rice cakes into the pan and fry for about 2 minutes on each side, until golden brown. Transfer the cakes to a clean piece of kitchen roll to remove any excess oil and repeat the process with the remaining oil and rice cakes.

Serve three rice cakes per person and top with the minty mango and a drizzle of maple syrup, if you like.

POST-WORKOUT
⇢MAKE AHEAD

AWESOME OVERNIGHT OATS

I'm obsessed with overnight oats and these certainly live up to their name. Easy to make and store, they are the perfect refuel meal and make life so much easier in the mornings.

⇢PREP 10 MINS,
PLUS SOAKING TIME

450ml almond milk
100g chocolate protein powder
60g blackberries, plus a few to garnish
40g blueberries, plus a few to garnish
60g honey
200g porridge oats

To serve
chopped hazelnuts
pumpkin seeds

Equipment
food processor

Place the almond milk, protein powder, blackberries, blueberries and honey into a food processor and blitz until smooth.

Pour the mixture over the porridge oats into a bowl, give it a stir and leave to soak for a minimum of 4 hours, but preferably overnight.

Serve the oats topped with a mixture of the berries, hazelnuts and pumpkin seeds.

POST-WORKOUT

BANGING BREAKFAST BURRITO

Mexicans have got it right by eating big burritos for breakfast. Ditch the sugary cereal and give this one a go. It's packed full of goodness and tastes banging.

➡**PREP 10 MINS**
➡**COOK 15 MINS**

1 x 415g tin of refried beans
large bunch of coriander, roughly chopped, plus 2 tbsp to garnish
½ tbsp coconut oil
1 red onion, finely sliced
2 jarred red peppers (about 100g), drained and cut into 1cm strips
½ tsp chilli flakes
275g thick-cut deli ham, sliced into 1cm chunks
small knob of butter
8 eggs, cracked and beaten
4 large tortillas
10 jarred jalapeño pepper pieces, roughly chopped

Tip the beans into a saucepan and add the coriander along with a small splash of water. Heat the beans slowly on the hob, stirring occasionally.

Meanwhile, melt the coconut oil in a large frying pan over a medium to high heat. When it is hot, add the red onion and fry for 1 minute. Add the red peppers, chilli flakes and ham, and continue to stir-fry for another minute.

Increase the heat to maximum and add the knob of butter. When it has melted, pour in the eggs and begin to stir slowly, as if you are making scrambled eggs. Reduce the heat a little if the mixture starts to stick to the pan.

When the eggs are nearly cooked, stop stirring and leave the base of the eggs to set and brown a little – this will take a couple of minutes.

Zap the tortillas in your microwave to heat them up.

Sprinkle the jalapeño all over the top of the eggs and then give them one last stir to break them up. Take the pan off the heat.

Spread a good amount of the refried beans across the base of your tortilla, top with the egg mix, sprinkle on a little of the reserved coriander and then roll up your burrito and get stuck in.

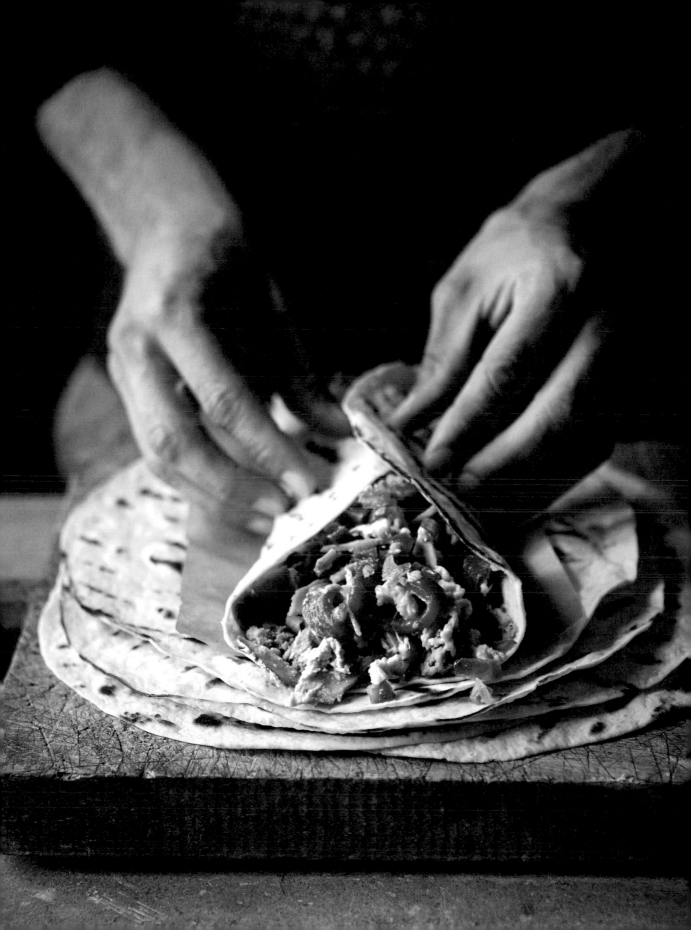

THE BODY COACH BRUNCH

This will make a perfect Sunday brunch for your family or friends. The truffle oil sounds a bit posh but it makes the poached eggs taste unreal. Don't worry if your eggs don't come out like they look in this picture – it has taken me years to poach the perfect egg!

➡PREP 10 MINS
➡COOK 10 MINS

4 eggs

4 drizzles of truffle oil

4 tsp chopped chives

250g asparagus, woody ends removed

4 thick slices of sourdough (or other good-quality bread)

4 slices of thick-cut deli ham

4 pinches of paprika, to serve

Bring two large saucepans of water to the boil.

Line up four ramekins or mugs and lay a piece of cling film over each one, leaving a large overhang on each. Push the cling flim into the base of the ramekin and then carefully crack an egg into each. Drizzle a little truffle oil and sprinkle a teaspoon of chives over each egg.

Gently draw up the overhanging sides of the cling film, twisting it and then tying a knot to get four wrapped eggs. Lower the eggs carefully into the first pan of water and poach for 4½ minutes.

While the eggs are poaching, boil the asparagus in the second pan of water for 3 minutes. Start toasting your bread, and, if you want to heat up your ham, lay it on a plate, cover it with cling film and zap in the microwave for 2 minutes.

To serve, place a slice of ham on each slice of toast. Use a pair of scissors to snip the cling film and peel a perfect poached egg from its wrapping. Place it on top of the ham.

Serve the asparagus on the side, ready to dip into the truffle-infused yolk. Give the whole thing a little sprinkle of paprika for an added kick.

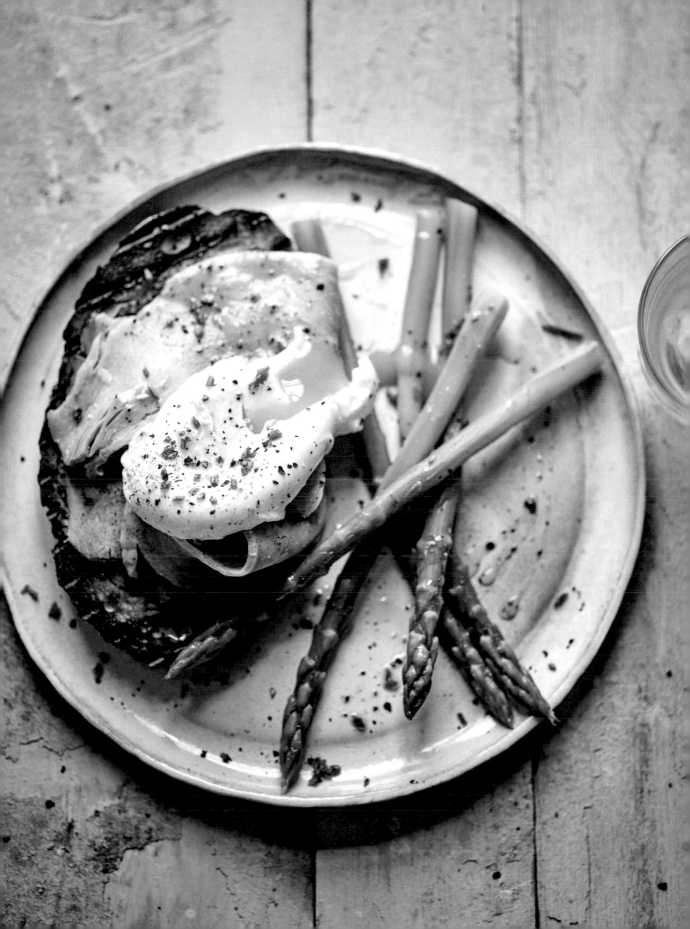

POST-WORKOUT

CHICKEN LINGUINE WITH FIERY RED-PEPPER SAUCE

Mmm . . . I love carbs! They make me so happy, especially after a good workout. This is probably the tastiest pasta sauce I've ever made – once you try it, you'll be making it again and again.

→ PREP 10 MINS
→ COOK 15 MINS

250g jarred red peppers, drained

2 cloves garlic, roughly chopped

1 tsp dried oregano

½ small bunch of basil, leaves only, roughly chopped

1 red chilli, finely sliced – and de-seeded if you don't like it hot

450g dried linguine

1 head of broccoli, florets only

1 medium courgette, cut into 1cm half moons

½ tbsp coconut oil

500g skinless chicken breast, cut into 1cm strips

salt and pepper

small bunch of parsley, roughly chopped, to serve

Equipment
food processor

Place the red peppers, garlic, oregano, basil and red chilli into a food processor and blitz until smooth. Set aside.

Bring a pan of water to the boil then cook your linguine according to packet instructions. Around 3 minutes before the pasta is cooked, remove about half a mug of cooking liquid from the pan and set it aside for later in the recipe.

Slide in the broccoli and courgette and continue to cook for the final 3 minutes, then drain the pasta and vegetables.

While the pasta is cooking, melt the oil in a large frying pan over a medium to high heat. When it is hot, add the chicken strips, season with salt and pepper and fry for about 5 minutes, or until just cooked through.

Add the pasta and vegetables directly into the pan with the chicken, and toss to combine. Add the pepper sauce and reserved cooking liquid to the pan, and stir again to mix everything together.

Season with salt and pepper, top with the chopped parsley and serve.

POST-WORKOUT

SPICY NOODLE SOUP

This is inspired by a dish I had on holiday called Laksa. It's basically a spicy fragrant coconut soup with chicken, prawn and noodles. You are going to love it.

⬦PREP 10 MINS
⬦COOK 15 MINS

½ tbsp coconut oil

3 star anise

3 lemongrass stalks, tender white parts only, finely sliced

5cm fresh ginger, roughly chopped into large chunks

4 bird's eye chillies

4 large shallots, finely sliced

zest and juice of 2 limes

500ml chicken stock

500ml coconut water

800g 'straight to wok' egg noodles

12 cooked prawns

300g cooked chicken, roughly shredded

4 boiled eggs, peeled and cut in half

2½ tbsp fish sauce

2 handfuls of beansprouts

small bunch of coriander, roughly chopped

Put on your kettle to boil.

Melt the coconut oil in a large saucepan over a medium to high heat. When it is hot, add the star anise, lemongrass, ginger, chillies, shallots and lime zest. Stir-fry the ingredients for 2 minutes.

Pour the chicken stock and coconut water into the pan and bring to the boil. Reduce the heat to a simmer for 2 minutes.

Tip the egg noodles into a colander and pour over the boiling water from the kettle. Carefully, using a fork or tongs, divide the warmed noodles between four bowls and then top each pile of noodles with three prawns, shredded chicken and one boiled egg.

Turn the heat off from under the hot stock and add the fish sauce and the lime juice. Carefully pour the hot liquid directly over the ingredients in the bowls and top with a handful of beansprouts and the coriander.

POST-WORKOUT

MISO RAMEN

This recipe not only tastes amazing it also looks the business. It's really filling, and so makes a great refuel meal after a HIIT session.

→**PREP 15 MINS**
→**COOK 15 MINS**

2 eggs

6 midget trees (tender-stem broccoli), trimmed

½ tbsp coconut oil

2 boneless and skinless chicken thighs, cut into 2cm strips

1 tbsp light soy sauce

2 tsp sesame oil

2 tsp honey

600ml chicken stock

50g brown rice miso

250g 'straight to wok' egg noodles

12 cooked prawns

2 spring onions, finely sliced

2 red shallots, finely sliced – optional

Bring a saucepan of water to the boil. Carefully lower in the eggs and cook for 7 minutes. When the eggs have had 5 minutes, drop in the midget trees and continue to cook for a further 2 minutes before draining through a sieve and cooling both the eggs and broccoli under cold running water.

While the eggs are boiling away, melt the coconut oil in a frying pan over a medium to high heat. When it is hot, add the chicken thigh strips and fry for 3–4 minutes or until they are just cooked through. Check by slicing into one of the larger pieces to make sure the meat is white all the way through, with no raw pink bits left.

When the chicken is cooked, pour in the soy sauce, sesame oil and honey, and heat until just starting to bubble. Turn off the heat and leave the chicken to one side.

Bring the chicken stock to the boil in a fresh pan and when just simmering, ladle a small amount out into a bowl. Splodge the miso into the bowl and give it a good stir to make sure it is fully dissolved. Pour the miso stock back into the pan and bring the liquid back up to the boil. Take the pan off the heat.

Divide the noodles between two bowls and then pour the hot stock over the top. Pile on the midget trees, cooked chicken, prawns, spring onions and red shallots, if you like. Peel the eggs, cut them in half and place them on top. Serve up and slurp down.

★ *YOU CAN TRANSPORT THIS BY PUTTING THE SOUP IN A FLASK AND ALL THE OTHER BITS IN A BOX. WHEN YOU ARE READY TO EAT, POUR OVER THE HOT STOCK, PING IT IN THE MICROWAVE FOR 1 MINUTE AND ENJOY.*

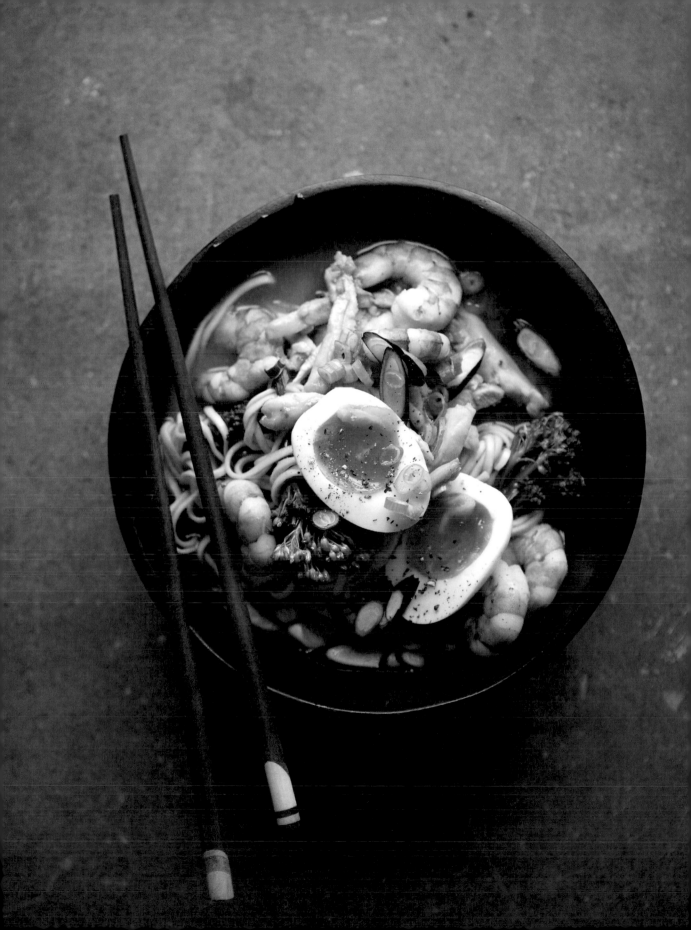

MINESTRONE SOUP

This is a really quick and easy meal to prepare and it's big enough to feed a family of four.

➡ PREP 15 MINS
➡ COOK 40 MINS

½ tbsp coconut oil

4 rashers of smoked back bacon, visible fat removed and cut into 1cm strips

2 cloves garlic, finely chopped

1 large onion, diced

2 celery sticks, diced

4 carrots, diced

2 potatoes, peeled and diced

1 x 400g tin of chopped tomatoes

1 x 400g tin of cannellini beans, drained and rinsed

200g orzo pasta

600ml fresh chicken stock

100g green beans, trimmed and cut into 2.5cm pieces

100g savoy cabbage leaves, shredded

small bunch of parsley, roughly chopped

Melt the coconut oil in a large saucepan over a medium to high heat. When it is melted, add the bacon and fry for 2 minutes, or just long enough for the bacon to take on a little colour.

Add the garlic, onion, celery, carrots and potatoes to the pan and fry, stirring occasionally for 5 minutes, until the mixture begins to soften.

Chuck in the chopped tomatoes, cannellini beans, orzo and 400ml of the chicken stock. Bring the whole lot slowly to the boil, stirring occasionally to ensure none of the vegetables stick to the bottom of the pan. Simmer the soup for 25–30 minutes, until all the ingredients are very soft.

Pour in the remaining 200ml of stock and add the green beans and shredded cabbage to the pan. Simmer for 5 more minutes.

Just before serving, stir through the chopped parsley.

POST-WORKOUT
→**LOW & SLOW**
→**GOOD TO FREEZE**

→**PREP 15 MINS**
→**COOK 1 HR 45 MINS**

1 tbsp olive oil

14 skinless chicken thighs, bone-in

3 carrots, diced into 2cm pieces

3 celery sticks, diced into 2cm pieces

2 onions, diced

2 sprigs of thyme

1 bay leaf

7cm fresh ginger, roughly chopped

200g macaroni (or other pasta)

salt and pepper

large bunch of parsley, finely chopped

ULTIMATE CHICKEN SOUP

This chicken soup requires a bit of patience but it's so worth the wait. It's high in protein and carbohydrates, which is just what you need after a workout.

Heat the oil in your largest saucepan over a medium to high heat. Fry the chicken thighs in 2–3 batches until browned, transferring them to a plate when they are ready.

Add the carrots, celery, onions, thyme, bay leaf and ginger to the pan and fry, stirring every now and then, for 5 minutes. Tip the chicken thighs back into the pan and generously cover the whole lot with about 3–4 litres of water.

Bring to a simmer, and as it comes to the boil, skim off the nasty solid stuff and fat that rise to the surface. It is worth skimming the soup a couple of times as it cooks to give you a reduced-fat, clear broth.

Simmer the soup, uncovered, for at least 1 hour 30 minutes. You can keep it boiling for anything up to 3 hours if you like, making sure you add a little water every now and then.

When the soup has had its cooking time, transfer the chicken thighs to a dish and leave until cool enough to handle. Tip the pasta into the soup and let it simmer away for 15 minutes or until cooked.

When the chicken is cool enough to handle, strip the meat from the bone, ripping it into pieces as you go. When the pasta is ready, tip the meat back into the soup, season generously with salt and pepper, and stir through the parsley. Serve.

PHAT FISH FINGER SANDWICH

Wow! Look at the state of that. That's what I call a fish finger sandwich. I mean, who wouldn't want to eat that after a workout?

➡**PREP 15 MINS**
➡**COOK 10 MINS**

4 x 130g boneless and skinless cod fillets

75g plain flour

2 eggs, beaten

200g fresh breadcrumbs

1 tbsp coconut oil

1½ tbsp zero-fat Greek yoghurt

juice of 1 lemon

2 tbsp chopped parsley

1 shallot, finely diced

2 large sub rolls

2 gherkins, sliced thinly lengthways

2 handfuls of watercress, to serve

Take each fillet of fish and cut it in half to make eight 'fingers'. Place the flour, beaten eggs and breadcrumbs into three separate bowls.

Pick up one fish finger and dip it into the flour, giving it a little shake to remove any excess. Dip the finger into the egg and then finally into the breadcrumbs. Repeat the process with all of the fish fingers.

It is likely that you will have to cook the fingers in two batches, so melt half of the oil in a large frying pan over a medium heat. When it is hot, gently lay the crumbed fish in the pan and fry for about 2 minutes on all four sides. Drain the cooked fingers on a clean piece of kitchen roll and repeat the cooking process with the remaining crumbed fingers.

While the second batch of fish is cooking, mix together the yoghurt, lemon juice, parsley and shallot. Spread the sauce thinly over the inside of the sub rolls.

When all the fish fingers are cooked, pile them into the sub rolls, top with the sliced gherkins and watercress, and chow down.

★ *YOU CAN SPICE UP YOUR FISH FINGERS BY ADDING GROUND SPICES SUCH AS PAPRIKA OR CUMIN TO THE FLOUR OR BREADCRUMBS.*

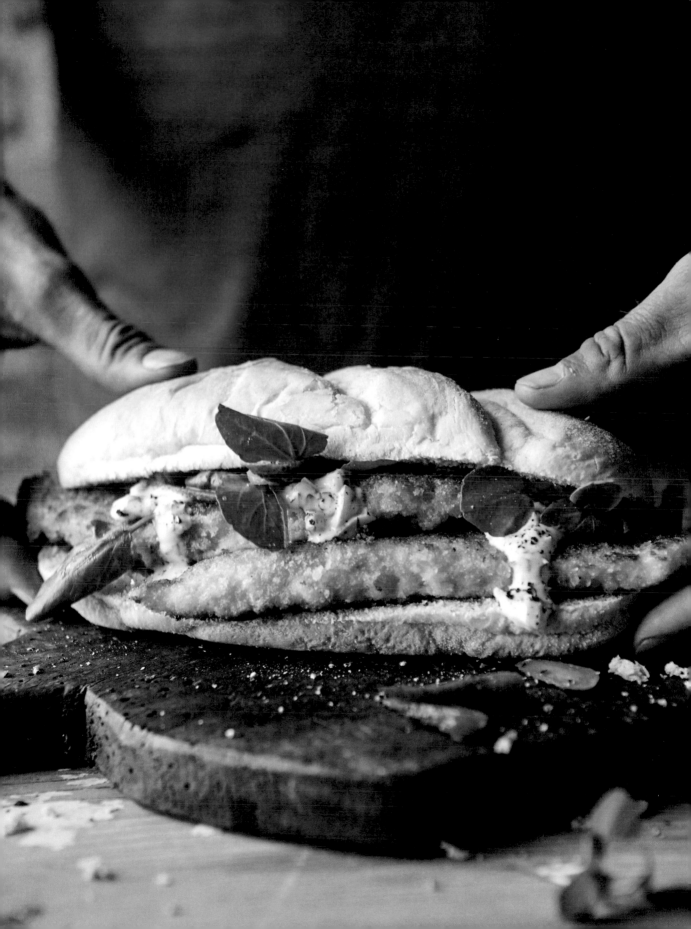

POST-WORKOUT

CHICKEN & LEEK GNOCCHI BAKE

Gnocchi is becoming my new favourite carb source. I can't work out if it's a potato or a pasta but I don't care because it tastes so good. The kids and adults will all enjoy this one.

➡ **PREP 15 MINS**
➡ **COOK 45 MINS**

500g fresh gnocchi
100g kale, hard stalks removed
1 chicken stock cube
½ tbsp coconut oil
1 tbsp butter
1 onion, diced
2 leeks, cut into 5mm rounds
500g skinless chicken breast, cut into 3cm chunks
200g mushrooms, brushed clean and roughly sliced
25g plain flour
½ tsp English mustard powder
25g parmesan, grated
½ bunch of parsley, roughly chopped
salt and pepper
3 tbsp fresh breadcrumbs
steamed vegetables, to serve – optional

Equipment
23 x 18cm baking dish

Bring a saucepan of water to the boil and preheat your oven to 190°C (fan 170°C/gas mark 5).

When the water is boiling, drop in the gnocchi and cook for 2 minutes, then add the kale and cook for a further 2 minutes. Use a mug to scoop out 300ml of the cooking liquid. Add the chicken stock cube into the mug, stir, and set aside. Drain the gnocchi and kale.

While the gnocchi is cooking, melt the coconut oil and butter in a large frying pan over a medium to high heat. When hot, add the chopped onion and leeks and fry for about 3 minutes, or until the vegetables begin to soften. Crank up the heat to maximum and add both the chicken and mushrooms to the pan. Stir-fry for a few minutes or until the meat takes on a little colour.

Reduce the heat to just below medium and stir in the flour. Stir-fry for 1 minute, then gradually start adding the stock. Stir in a quarter of the liquid at a time to avoid lumps.

When all of the liquid has been added, bring to the boil, then take the pan off the heat and stir in the mustard powder, parmesan and chopped parsley. Season with salt and pepper.

Tip the drained gnocchi and kale into the pan and gently stir everything together. Tip the mixture into a baking dish, sprinkle the breadcrumbs all over the top and then slide it into the oven. Bake for 20 minutes or until the breadcrumbs are golden.

Remove the dish from the oven and serve on its own or with a big bowl of steamed vegetables.

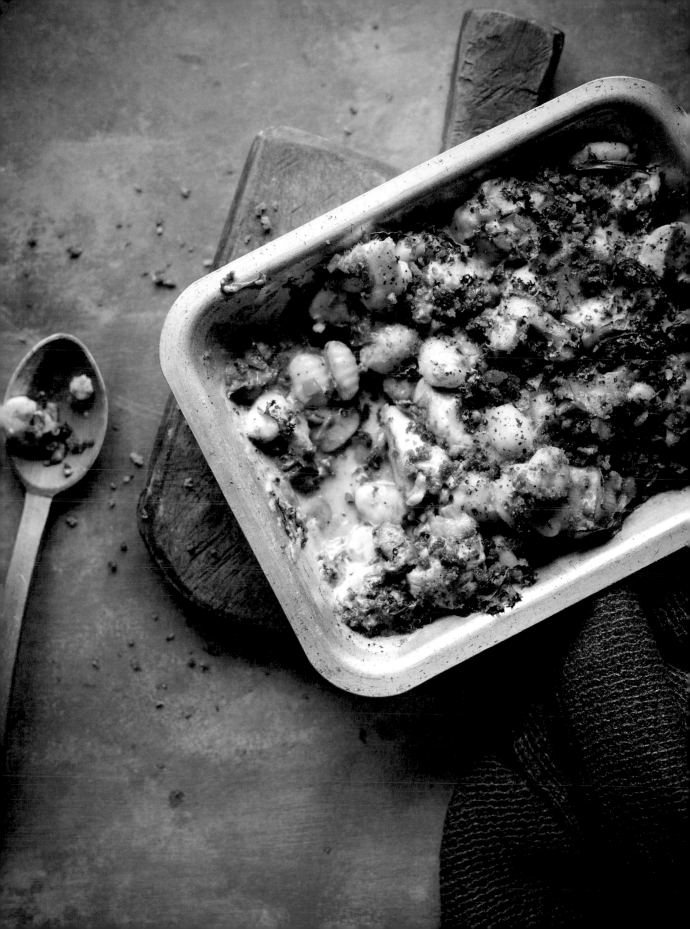

POST-WORKOUT
→BBQ

LAMB MCLEANIE BURGER

If you follow me on social media you'll know that burgers are my favourite thing in the world. This one, made with lamb mince and breadcrumbs, is a real winner.

→**PREP 15 MINS**
→**COOK 50 MINS**

750g new or Charlotte potatoes, cut in half lengthways
1 tbsp olive oil
1 tsp smoked paprika
salt and pepper
2 tsp coconut oil
1 red onion, diced
2 cloves garlic, finely chopped
½ cucumber
800g reduced-fat lamb mince
2 tsp ground cumin, plus an extra pinch
50g fresh breadcrumbs
1 egg
150g zero-fat Greek yoghurt

To serve
6 burger buns
chipotle paste
sliced tomato and lettuce leaves

Preheat your oven to 180°C (fan 160°C/gas mark 4). Fire up the barbecue or preheat the griddle pan.

Chuck the potatoes into a roasting dish, pour over the oil, sprinkle on the paprika and season with salt and pepper. Toss the whole lot together so the potatoes are evenly slicked in the oil, then slide into the oven and roast for 45 minutes, turning a couple of times during the cooking process.

Melt the coconut oil in a frying pan over a medium to high heat. When it is hot, add the onion and cook for 2 minutes, stirring regularly. Next, add the garlic to the pan and continue to fry for 1 more minute. Tip the mixture onto a plate and leave to cool a little.

Grate the cucumber and place it into a sieve. Sprinkle over ½ teaspoon of salt, mix well and leave the cucumber to sit and drain while you carry on with the rest of the recipe.

Plonk the mince into a large bowl and add the 2 teaspoons of ground cumin, breadcrumbs and egg along with some salt and pepper. Scrape in the onion and garlic and then use your hands to mix the whole lot together.

With slightly damp hands, shape the meat into six roughly equal-sized burgers. Cook the burgers on the barbecue or a griddle pan for about 4 minutes on each side, then remove from the heat and leave to rest for a couple of minutes.

Give the draining cucumbers a squeeze, then tip them into a bowl with the yoghurt, season with salt and pepper and the final pinch of ground cumin, and mix well with a spoon.

Build your burger however you like. I prefer to spread the bun with chipotle paste, whack on the burger, top with tomatoes and lettuce, dollop with the cucumber yoghurt and serve with the paprika spuds.

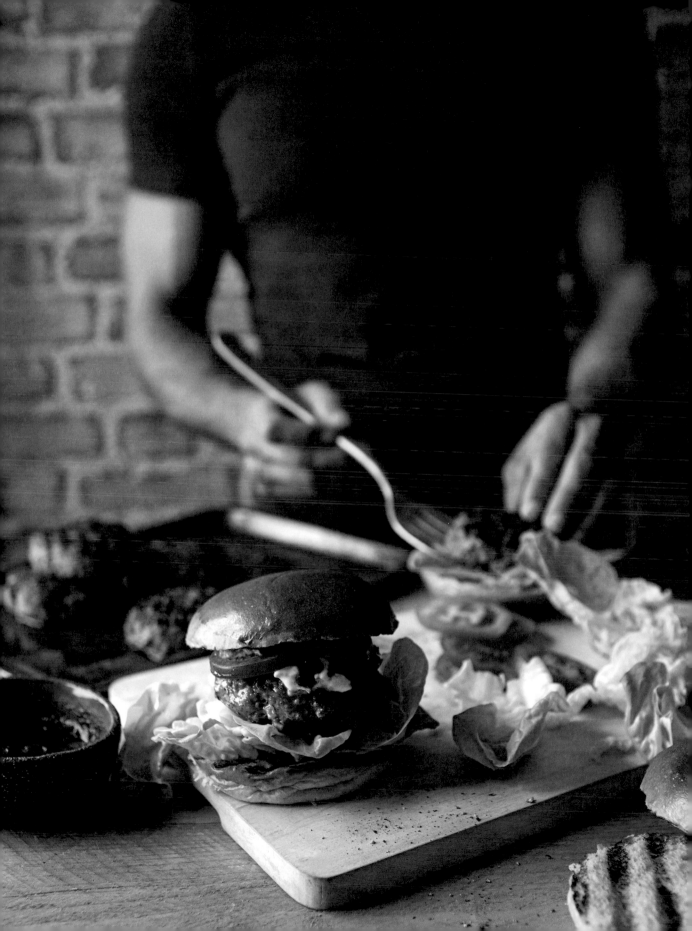

Serves 2

POST-WORKOUT

SMOKEY JOE'S PIZZA

Next time you fancy a pizza night, give this one a try instead of ordering a greasy takeaway – it's so much healthier and tastier. Making the dough yourself is easy and you will feel proud when you sit down to eat your very own handmade pizza.

**▶ PREP 25 MINS,
   PLUS PROVING TIME
▶ COOK 15–20 MINS**

1 x 7g sachet of fast-action yeast
250g strong flour, plus a little extra for rolling
salt
40g semolina

For the topping
115g baby spinach
125g kidney beans, drained and rinsed
1 x 400g tin of chopped tomatoes
50g barbecue sauce
150g cooked chicken, torn into strips
2 eggs

First, make the dough by placing the yeast into a jug and pouring over 150ml of warm water. Whisk together.

Tip the flour into a large bowl and add a good pinch of salt. Pour the yeast mixture into the flour and use a fork or a wooden spoon to bring it together. When the ingredients are roughly combined, generously dust a clean work surface with flour and tip the dough onto it.

Now knead the dough for about 5 minutes. You can do this any way you want, but I find that a mixture of pounding, folding and squeezing seems to work well. The dough should become elastic with all the ingredients fully combined. Bring the dough into a ball shape, place in a large bowl, cover with cling film and leave in a warm place to prove for 1 hour 30 minutes.

When you are ready to cook the pizza, preheat your oven to 220°C (fan 200°C/gas mark 7).

Tip the dough out of the bowl and 'knock it back', which means kneading it again for a couple of minutes until the air is worked out of it. ➡

★ *YOUR PIZZA DOUGH MIGHT FEEL A LITTLE WET TO BEGIN WITH. FLOUR YOUR SURFACE WELL AND PERSEVERE WITH THE KNEADING AND IT WILL COME TOGETHER – THE WETTER THE DOUGH, THE BETTER THE PIZZA.*

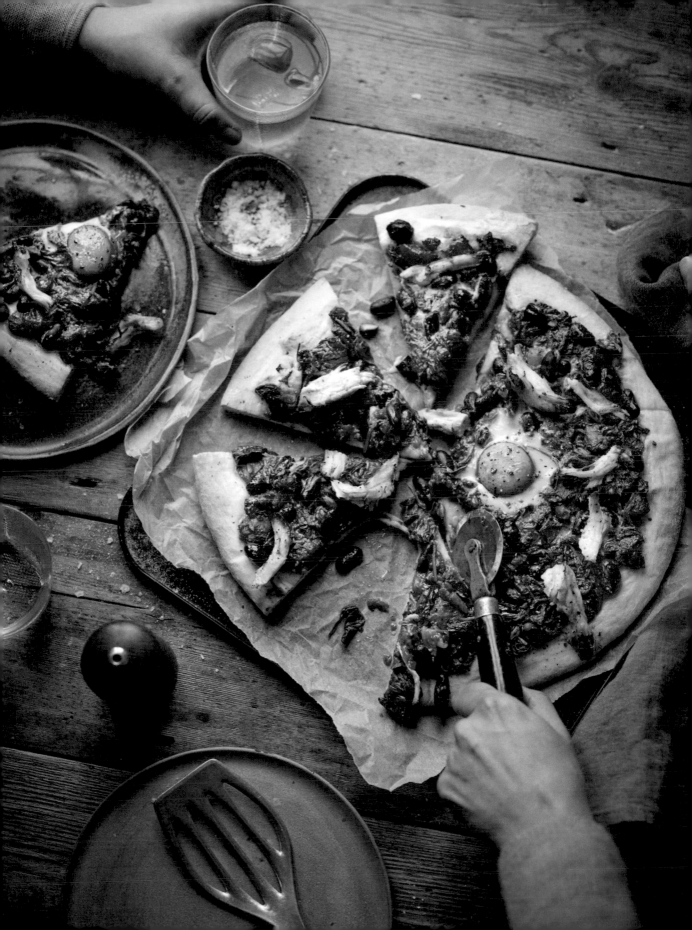

SMOKEY JOE'S PIZZA (CONTINUED)

Dust a clean surface with flour and roll out the dough to a circle of even thickness, slightly thicker than a pound coin. Scatter the semolina onto a flat baking tray and carefully move your rolled dough onto it – don't worry if the pizza loses a bit of shape, just push it out with your hands.

Next, make the topping. Tip the spinach leaves into a large colander and pour over boiling water to wilt them. Then rinse the spinach under cold running water until it is cool enough to handle, and give it a good squeeze to remove as much liquid as possible. Put the spinach into a bowl with the kidney beans.

Tip the chopped tomatoes into a sieve, give them a shake to remove a good amount of the liquid, and then tip the leftover tomato into the bowl with the spinach and kidney beans. Pour in the barbecue sauce and mix the ingredients together.

Spread the mixture evenly over the pizza base, leaving two little indents in the centre. Scatter the chicken all over the mix and then carefully crack an egg into each hole.

Cook the pizza in the oven for 15–20 minutes, until the egg whites are set, but the yolks are still runny. Serve immediately.

GINGER CHICKEN BIRIYANI

Did someone say curry night? I hope so. If you want to impress your mates, don't order one in, get this one going instead. It tastes authentic and is leaner than any takeaway.

→PREP 15 MINS
→COOK 50 MINS

2 tbsp coconut oil

6 cloves

5 cardamom pods, lightly crushed

2 onions, roughly chopped

7cm fresh ginger, finely chopped

5 cloves garlic, finely chopped

1 tbsp garam masala

2 tsp ground coriander

2 tsp ground ginger

1 tsp ground turmeric

1½ tsp chilli powder – more if you like it hot

10 boneless and skinless chicken thighs, roughly cut into 4cm chunks

3 large tomatoes, roughly chopped

2 bunches of fresh coriander, roughly chopped

3 x 250g packets of pre-cooked rice

pomegranate seeds, to serve

Equipment
food processor
large hob-proof casserole dish

Melt 1½ tablespoons of the coconut oil in a large saucepan over a medium to high heat. When it is hot, add the cloves and cardamom pods and fry for 2 minutes. While the spices are frying, blitz the onions in a food processor until they are pretty much smooth and tip straight into the pan.

Fry the onions and spices, stirring regularly for about 8 minutes, until soft. Add the fresh ginger and garlic and continue to cook for another 2 minutes, then sprinkle in all of the ground herbs and spices. Fry, stirring constantly for 1 minute. If the mixture is starting to stick to the bottom of the pan, pour in a little water.

Scrape in the chicken and stir, cooking for another minute or so. Next add the chopped tomatoes and pour in 200ml of water. Gently bring the whole lot to a simmer. Simmer the curry with a cocked lid on top for 30 minutes, giving it a little stir every now and then to make sure it isn't burning at the bottom of the pan.

After 30 minutes, take the curry off the heat and stir through half of the chopped coriander. Leave the curry to cool to room temperature.

About 15 minutes before you are ready to eat, zap the rice in the microwave. Melt the remaining coconut oil in a large casserole pan and carefully tilt the pan so that the bottom and the sides are greased with coconut oil. Remove the pan from the heat. ➡

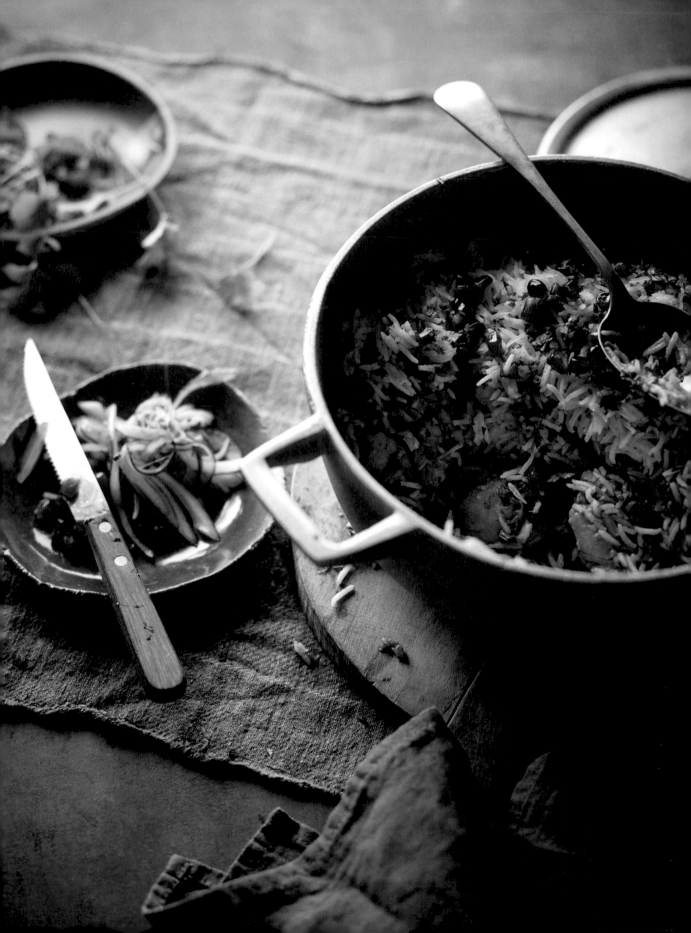

GINGER CHICKEN BIRIYANI

Take one packet of rice and tip it into the bottom of the pan, using a spoon or fork to spread it out roughly. Next, spoon half of the curry straight onto the rice and spread it out evenly. Tip the second packet of rice onto the curry and spread it over evenly, then pour the remaining curry onto the rice. Spread it out and then cover with the final packet of rice.

Place the lid tightly on top and put the casserole over a low heat for 5 minutes. The rice at the bottom of the pan should have browned a little and turned crunchy.

Proudly carry your curry to the table, remove the lid and top with the remaining chopped coriander and pomegranate seeds.

★ *IF YOU DON'T HAVE A POT WITH A TIGHT LID, LAY A CLEAN TEA TOWEL OVER THE TOP OF THE PAN AND THEN PLACE A LID, PLATE OR BAKING TRAY OVER THE TOP. BE CAREFUL TO TUCK IN THE ENDS OF THE TEA TOWEL SO THEY DON'T CATCH FIRE!*

POST-WORKOUT
- **LOW & SLOW**
- **GOOD TO FREEZE**

NANNY KATH'S BEEF STEW

Hold tight for my Nan's secret stew recipe. She used to make me this for me when I was growing up and I promised her that when I wrote a friends and family book I would include it. I truly love this recipe and I'm so happy to be sharing it with you.

- **PREP 15 MINS**
- **COOK 2 HRS 45 MINS**

3 tbsp olive oil

1 large onion, diced

1 large carrot, diced

2 celery sticks, diced

1 star anise

1½ tsp ground ginger

1 bay leaf

3 sprigs of thyme

275g tomatoes, roughly chopped into large chunks

750ml beef stock

1.5kg beef shin, cut into 3cm chunks

2 large potatoes, peeled and cut into fifths

buttered greens and carrots, to serve

For the dumplings

125g self-raising flour

125g suet

large bunch of parsley, roughly chopped

salt and pepper

Equipment

large hob-proof casserole dish or ovenproof saucepan

Heat 1 tablespoon of the oil in the casserole dish or saucepan over a medium to high heat. When it is hot, slide in the onion, carrot and celery and fry, stirring occasionally for 8 minutes, by which time the vegetables will have softened a little.

Drop in the star anise, ground ginger, bay leaf and thyme sprigs. Stir-fry for a further 2 minutes. Add the tomatoes and keep frying for about 5 minutes, until the tomatoes start to collapse – reduce the heat a little if they start to burn.

When the tomatoes have collapsed, pour in 500ml of the stock and allow it to come slowly up to the boil, then lower the heat to a simmer.

Heat 1 more tablespoon of the oil in a large frying pan over a high heat. When it is hot, add half of the beef shin chunks. Do not move the meat; simply allow it to colour for 2 minutes. Flip the meat over and brown on the second side for another 2 minutes. When the meat is golden brown all over, tip it straight into the simmering casserole dish. Repeat the process with the last of the oil and the remaining beef.

Simmer the beef with a cocked lid on top for 90 minutes, until meltingly tender.

When the beef has about 10 minutes to go, add the potatoes to the casserole dish and top up with a little more stock if you think it's needed. Preheat your oven to 180°C (fan 160°C/gas mark 4) and prepare the dumplings. Tip the self-raising flour and suet into a bowl along with the chopped parsley and a good pinch of salt and pepper. Make a small well in the middle and pour in 100ml of water. ➡

★ *IF YOU DON'T LIKE THE FLAVOUR OF SUET, THEN YOU CAN JUST SWAP IT FOR BUTTER.*

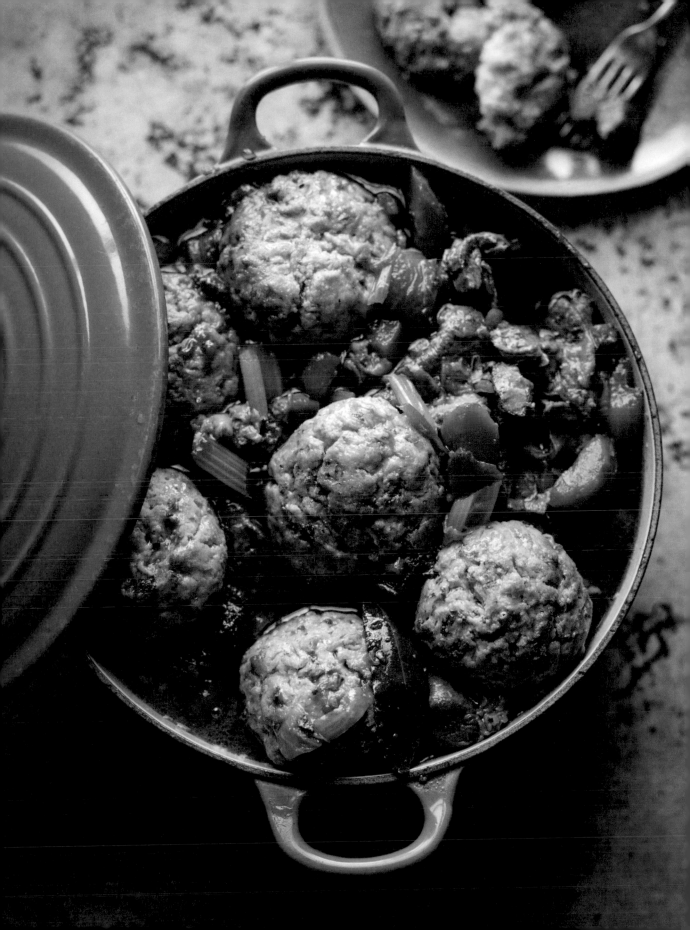

Gradually incorporate the flour and suet mixture into the liquid to form a pliable dough that holds its shape. You may need to add a little more water if it's too dry.

Roll the dough into eight equal-sized balls. When the beef is tender, drop the dumplings directly into the stew, leaving a decent space between each one.

Once all the dumplings are in the stew, put the lid on top and slide the whole casserole dish or pan into the oven. Bake with the lid on for 35 minutes.

Take the casserole out of the oven and remove the lid to reveal your puffed-up dumplings. Spoon a little liquid over each one and slide the casserole back into the oven for 10 minutes, until the dumplings have a lovely gloss.

Serve up your stew with buttered greens and carrots.

SUSHI RICE CHICKEN BOWL

This is a really tasty recipe that I think you'll love. Sushi rice can be found in most supermarkets now, and is actually very easy to cook.

►PREP 15 MINS, PLUS SOAKING TIME
►COOK 30 MINS

400g sushi rice
1 tbsp coconut oil
2 cloves garlic
400g skinless chicken breast, cut into 1cm strips
2 tsp light soy sauce
½ tbsp honey
200g green beans, trimmed
250g baby spinach
2 tsp sesame oil
1½ tbsp rice wine vinegar
½ tsp sugar
1 tsp salt

To serve
4 fried eggs
chilli flakes

Cover the rice with cold water and leave it to sit for 15 minutes. Drain the rice in a sieve and rinse for about 30 seconds under cold running water. Tip the drained rice into a saucepan and then cover with 400ml of water.

Put the saucepan onto the hob and bring to the boil over a high heat. Simmer for about 1 minute, then clamp on a lid and reduce the heat to minimum. Leave the rice to cook for 12 minutes, then turn off the heat completely and let the rice sit with the lid on for a further 5 minutes. At no point during the cooking process should you stir the rice or remove the lid to have a sneak peek.

While the rice is cooking, bring another saucepan of water to the boil and melt the coconut oil in a frying pan over a medium to high heat. Finely chop one of the garlic cloves and add it to the hot oil, followed quickly by the chicken strips. Stir-fry the chicken for about 5 minutes, or until it is cooked through. Check by slicing into one of the larger pieces to make sure the meat is white all the way through, with no raw pink bits left. Pour in the soy sauce and honey and stir.

When the saucepan of water is boiling, drop in the green beans and simmer for 3 minutes. Meanwhile, put the spinach into a colander and when the beans are cooked, drain them directly over the spinach. The heat from the boiling water should be enough to wilt the spinach. ➡

Rinse the beans and spinach under cold running water until cool enough to handle, then give them a squeeze to remove the excess water.

Put them into a bowl and grate the remaining garlic clove over the top. Pour in the sesame oil and toss together until combined.

Pour the rice vinegar into a bowl and stir in the sugar and salt. Lift the lid off the steaming rice and pour over the vinegar mixture, using a fork to stir it in.

Portion out your rice, top with the chicken, vegetables and a fried egg each, and sprinkle with chilli flakes.

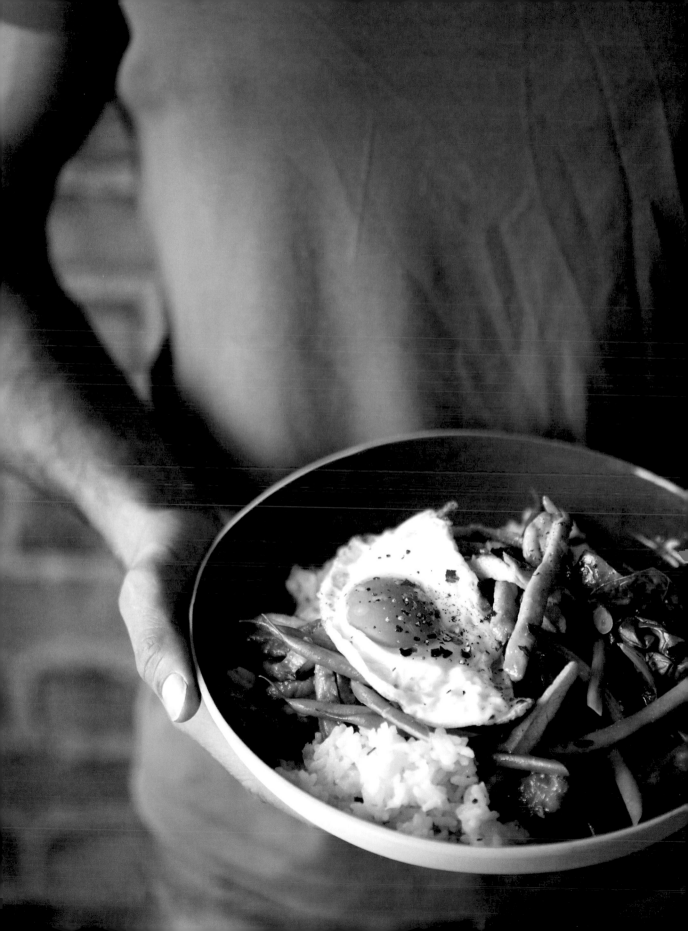

SWEET POTATO SHAKSHUKA

This makes a really great meal or breakfast for any day of the week. I use sweet potato and ham in this recipe, and they taste incredible.

◆PREP 10 MINS
◆COOK 20 MINS

2 sweet potatoes, peeled and cut into 2cm chunks

½ tbsp coconut oil

4 red onions, sliced

1 tsp chilli flakes – more if you like it hot

10 sage leaves, finely sliced

200g kale, stalks removed

275g thick-cut deli ham, cut into 1cm strips

1 x 400g tin of chopped tomatoes

4 eggs

large bunch of parsley, roughly chopped

Place the sweet potato chunks into a bowl along with a splash of water. Cover with cling film, zap in the microwave for 4 minutes and then leave until ready to use.

While the sweet potatoes are spinning, melt the coconut oil in a large saucepan over a medium to high heat. When it is hot, add the sliced onions and cook for 3 minutes until starting to soften. Sprinkle in the chilli flakes and sliced sage leaves and continue to stir-fry for 2 minutes.

Unwrap the sweet potatoes, drain off the excess water and then chuck them into the pan. Pile in the kale and keep stirring until it wilts – this will take about 5 minutes.

Stir in the ham strips, then pour in the chopped tomatoes along with half a tin of water. Bring to the boil. One at a time, make a small indent in the mixture with a wooden spoon and crack an egg into each one.

Place a lid on top and cook for 7 minutes, or until the eggs are cooked to your liking. Sprinkle with the chopped parsley and serve.

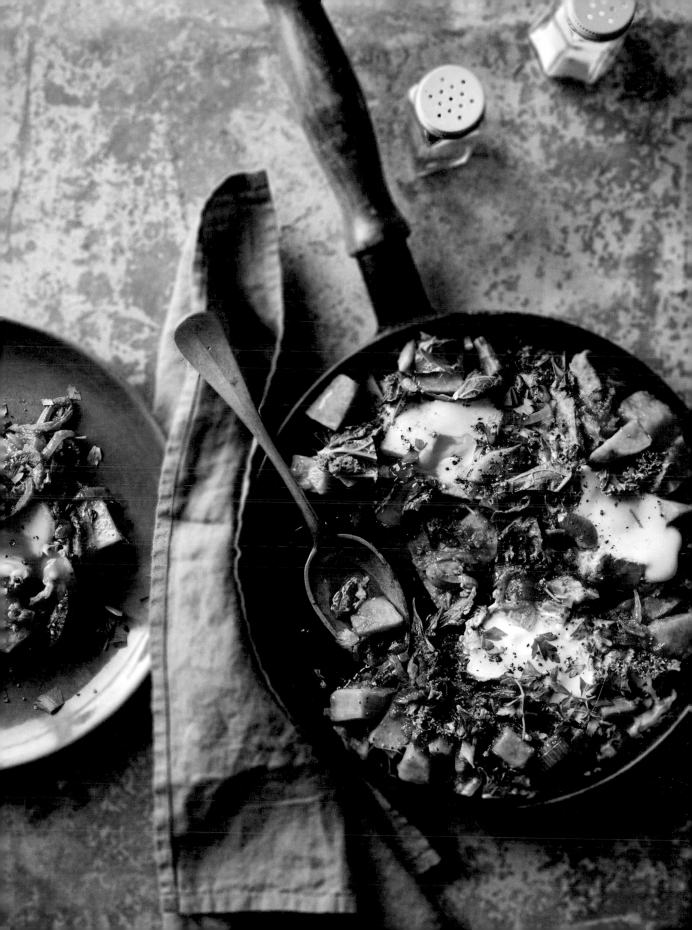

PRAWN & QUINOA FRITTERS

Sweet and nutty, prawns and quinoa work perfectly together in fritters. Once you try these you'll definitely be making them again.

→ PREP 10 MINS
→ COOK 15 MINS

1 medium courgette, grated
5 spring onions, finely sliced
100g pre-cooked quinoa
2 red chillies, de-seeded and finely chopped
300g raw prawns, peeled, cleaned and roughly cut into small pieces
½ tsp ground turmeric
1 tsp paprika
75g plain flour
1 egg
1 tbsp coconut oil

To serve
sweet chilli sauce
big green salad

Place all of the ingredients apart from the oil and chilli sauce into a bowl and mix until well combined.

Heat a large frying pan over a medium to high heat and add a little coconut oil. When the oil has melted and is hot, dollop about 2 tablespoons of the mixture into the pan, spreading it out until about 1cm thick. I can normally fit three fritters into a pan at once, but this will depend on the size of your pan.

Fry the fritters for 2–3 minutes on each side until dark golden and crisp at the edges.

When the fritters are cooked, slide them out and onto a clean piece of kitchen roll to blot off any excess oil.

Repeat the process with the remaining mixture and then serve up with the sweet chilli sauce and a big green salad.

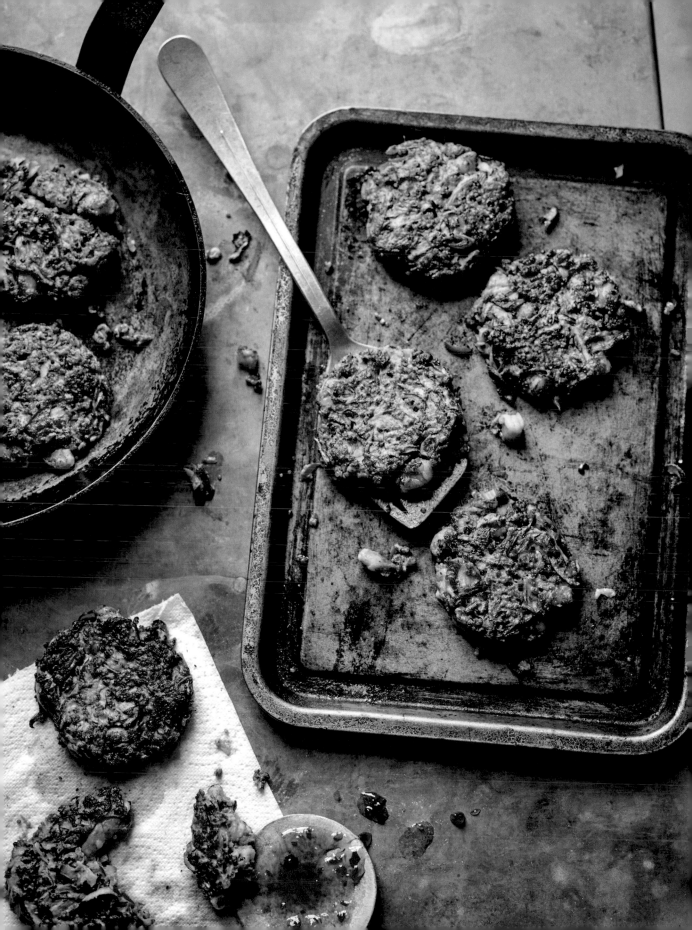

**POST-WORKOUT
→GOOD TO FREEZE**

MY FILIPINO CURRY

With sweet and sour flavours, this curry from the Philippines makes a nice change to traditional Indian or Asian curries.

**→PREP 15 MINS
→COOK 55 MINS**

1½ tbsp coconut oil

10 skinless chicken thighs, bone-in

2 red onions, diced

4 whole cloves

2 cinnamon sticks

3 cloves garlic, roughly chopped

2 red chillies, de-seeded and finely sliced

1 tsp ground ginger

1 tsp ground coriander

2 tsp red wine vinegar

200ml chicken stock

2 x 400g tins of kidney beans, drained and rinsed

large bunch of fresh coriander, roughly chopped

rice, to serve

Melt a little of the coconut oil in a large saucepan or hob-proof casserole dish over a high heat and add five of the chicken thighs. Brown the meat all over and then remove to a plate. Melt a little more oil in the same pan and fry the remaining five chicken thighs until golden brown all over, then remove those to a plate as well.

Dollop the remaining coconut oil into the pan and melt over a medium heat. Add the chopped onions, cloves, cinnamon sticks, garlic and red chillies and stir-fry for 5 minutes, or until the vegetables are beginning to soften.

Sprinkle in the ground ginger and coriander and stir in well. Increase the heat to maximum and pour in the vinegar, letting it bubble up and all but evaporate.

Slide the chicken thighs back into the pan and pour in the chicken stock. Bring to the boil, put a lid on and simmer for 35 minutes, or until the chicken is fully cooked and starting to fall off the bone.

Remove the lid and stir in the kidney beans. Bring the curry back up to the boil and simmer for 5 minutes before stirring through the chopped coriander and serving with bowls of steaming rice.

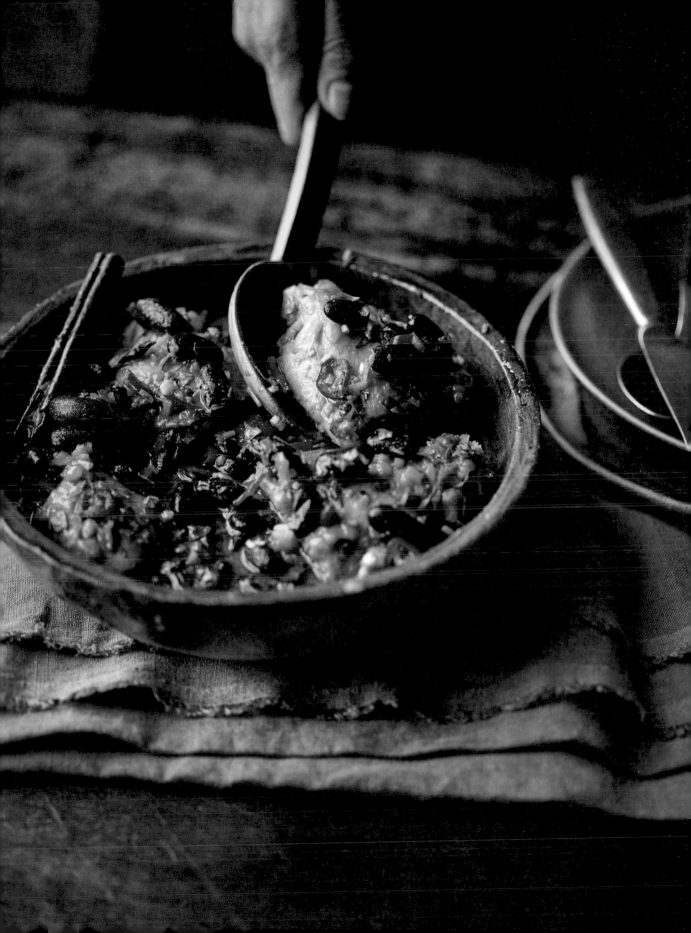

Serves 4

POST-WORKOUT
➧LOW & SLOW

➧**PREP 10 MINS**
➧**COOK 1 HR 45 MINS**

4 baking potatoes
1 tbsp sunflower oil
8 eggs
8 slices of thick-cut deli ham

To serve
baked beans
small salad – optional

CLASSIC HAM, EGG & 'CHIPS'

You can't beat a good family favourite, so I've made this healthier version of ham, eggs and chips. It's a classic that everyone is going to love, including the kids.

Preheat your oven to 180°C (fan 160°C/gas mark 4).

Use a pastry brush to brush each potato in turn with a little bit of oil. Place the oiled potatoes onto a baking tray. Slide it into the oven and bake for 1 hour 30 minutes, turning them once halfway through. The potatoes should be crisp and golden on the outside and soft and fluffy in the middle.

When the potatoes are ready, remove them from the oven but keep the oven on. When they are cool enough to handle, cut each one in half lengthways. Use a spoon to remove enough potato to make a deep narrow indent from the centre of each potato half. Crack an egg into each indent and then bake the potatoes for a further 12 minutes, until the the egg whites and yolks still have a little wobble to them.

While the eggs are baking, lay the ham slices onto a plate, pour over a little water, cover with cling film and zap in the microwave for 6–8 minutes on maximum power until the meat is heated through. Heat up your baked beans at this point too.

Serve up the ham, potatoes and eggs and beans.

★ *IF YOU PRICK THE POTATOES WITH A FORK AND ZAP THEM FOR 5 MINUTES IN THE MICROWAVE BEFORE THEY GO INTO THE OVEN, YOU CAN REDUCE THEIR COOKING TIME BY AROUND 45 MINUTES.*

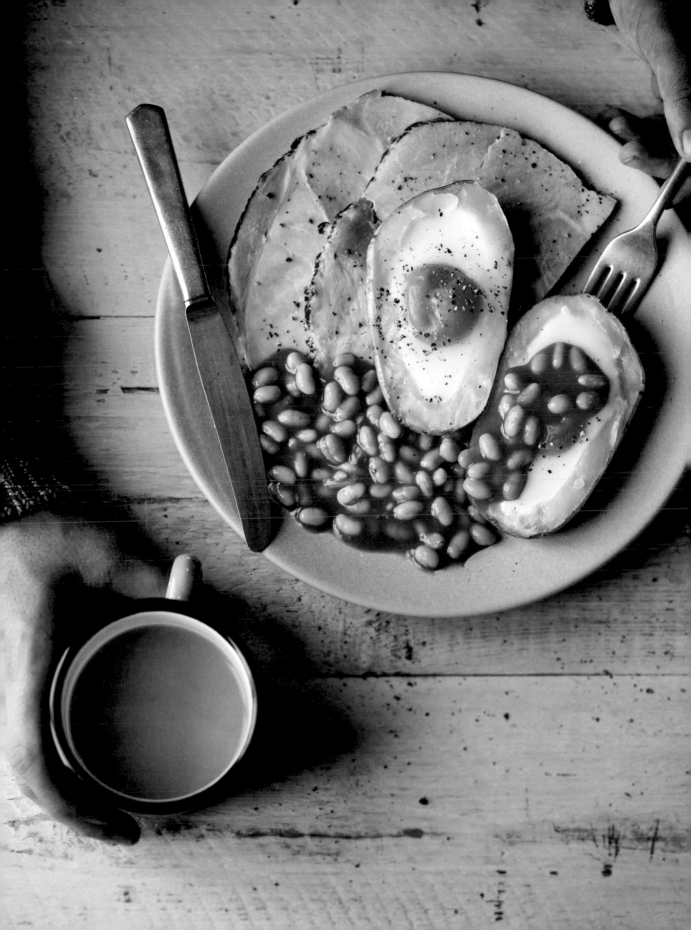

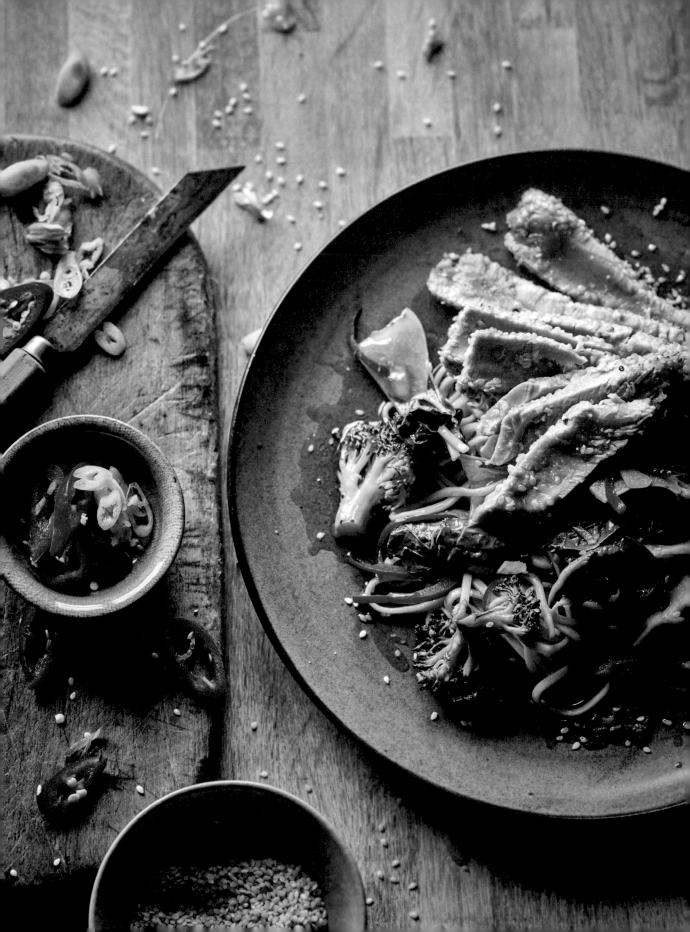

ASIAN STIR-FRY WITH SESAME TUNA

This is my favourite quick and easy stir-fry recipe. It's really simple to make and has so many flavours going on.

⇨PREP 10 MINS
⇨COOK 10 MINS

1½ tbsp sesame seeds

4 x 200g tuna steaks

salt

1 tbsp coconut oil

150g midget trees (tender-stem broccoli), any bigger stalks sliced in half lengthways

4 pak choy, roots cut off and leaves separated

4 spring onions, finely sliced

2 cloves garlic, finely chopped

150g oyster mushrooms, large ones roughly torn into halves or thirds

2 tbsp shaoxing wine

600g fresh egg noodles

1 tbsp light soy sauce

2 tsp sesame oil

2 red chillies, de-seeded and finely sliced

Scatter the sesame seeds over both sides of the tuna steaks, pushing them in a bit with your hands if they don't stick. The idea isn't to totally cover the tuna steaks, but to season them. Sprinkle with a little salt and leave to one side.

Melt half of the coconut oil in a large frying pan or wok over a high heat. When it is hot, carefully lay in the tuna steaks. Fry them for 2 minutes on each side for a rare steak. If you don't have a big enough frying pan, then cook the steaks in two batches. Slide the cooked steaks onto a plate to rest while you continue with the recipe.

Wipe out the frying pan using a clean piece of kitchen roll. Melt the remaining oil in the frying pan. When it is hot, chuck in the midget trees and pak choy and stir-fry for 1 minute – don't stir too much, because a bit of browned greens is very tasty. Add the spring onions, garlic and oyster mushrooms to the pan and stir-fry for about 2 minutes before pouring in the shaoxing wine.

Drop in the noodles and toss to mix with all the other ingredients. Pour in about 2 tablespoons of water. When the noodles are heated through, take the pan off the heat and stir in the soy sauce, sesame oil and sliced chillies.

Divvy up the noodles between four plates and top each one with a perfectly juicy tuna steak.

POST-WORKOUT

BAKED RISOTTO WITH COD

I'm totally obsessed with risotto at the moment. This one with cod and loads of veg is super healthy and really easy to prepare.

→PREP 10 MINS
→COOK 30 MINS

2 tbsp olive oil
1 onion, diced
1 leek, finely chopped
5 rashers of back bacon, visible fat removed, cut into 1cm strips
2 cloves garlic, finely chopped
200g chestnut mushrooms, sliced
1 tbsp tomato puree
2 tsp smoked sweet paprika
250g arborio or similar risotto rice
750ml chicken stock
6 x 150g skinless cod fillets
salt and pepper
16 cherry tomatoes, on the vine if possible

To serve
bunch of parsley, roughly chopped
lemon wedges

Equipment
large hob-proof casserole dish or ovenproof saucepan

Preheat your oven to 180°C (fan 160°C/gas mark 4).

Heat half of the olive oil in a large, hob-proof casserole dish or ovenproof saucepan over a medium to high heat. Slide in the onion, leek and sliced bacon and fry, stirring occasionally for 4 minutes, or until the onions and leek are starting to soften. Add the chopped garlic and mushrooms and continue to stir-fry for 2 minutes.

Squeeze in the tomato puree and stir through the mixture. Add the paprika and the rice and continue stir-frying for 30 seconds. Pour in the stock and bring to the boil, before clamping on a tight lid and transferring to the preheated oven. Bake the rice for 12 minutes.

While the rice is cooking, heat up half the remaining oil in a large frying pan over a high heat. Season the cod with salt and pepper and when the oil is hot, carefully lay three fillets in. Brown on both sides – you are not trying to cook the fish through here, just to brown it. Remove the browned cod to a plate and repeat the process with the remaining oil and fish.

After 12 minutes, take the risotto from the oven, remove the lid and give the rice a good stir. Lay the fish and tomatoes on top of the rice and then slide the dish back into the oven, uncovered. Roast the whole lot for 10 minutes, until the fish is perfectly cooked through and the tomatoes are softening but still holding their shape.

Remove the risotto from the oven, sprinkle with parsley and serve up with the lemon wedges.

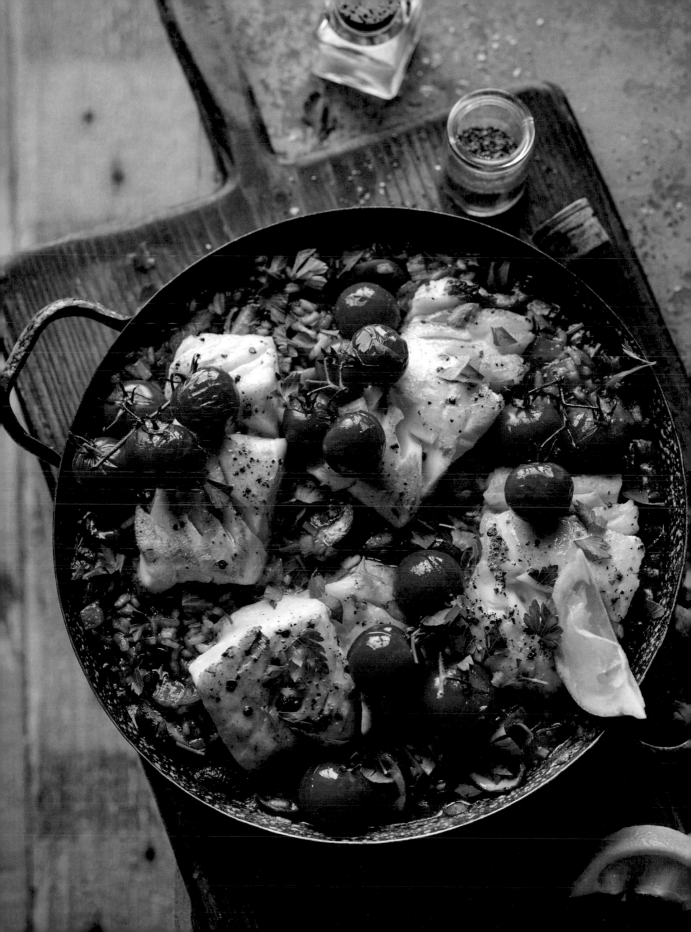

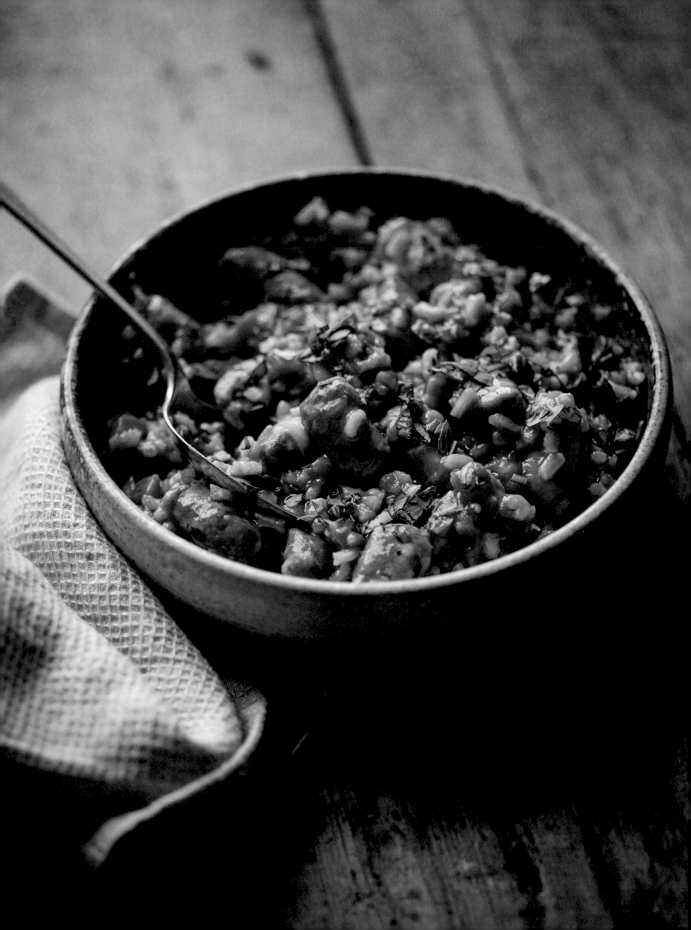

BAKED CHICKEN SAUSAGE RISOTTO

I told you I was obsessed with risotto, didn't I? Here's another absolute worldie. Baking risotto is much easier as it only requires a few stirs and the oven does the rest of the hard work.

▶PREP 10 MINS
▶COOK 35 MINS

1 tbsp coconut oil
1 red onion, diced
1 large carrot, diced
2 celery sticks, diced
1 red pepper, diced
2 sprigs of rosemary
8 chicken sausages, roughly chopped
300g arborio or similar risotto rice
1 x 400g tin chopped tomatoes
500ml chicken stock
large bunch of basil, roughly chopped

Equipment
large hob-proof casserole dish or ovenproof saucepan

Preheat your oven to 180°C (fan 160°C/gas mark 4).

Place a large, hob-proof casserole dish or ovenproof saucepan over a medium to high heat and add the coconut oil.

When the oil is melted and hot, chuck in the chopped red onion, carrot, celery and red pepper and cook, stirring regularly for 5 minutes or until the vegetables just begin to soften.

Increase the heat to maximum and push the frying vegetables to one side to leave a clear space in the pan. Drop the rosemary and the sausages into the gap and fry until you have some colour on the sausages.

Reduce the heat to medium and tip in the rice, gently and carefully stirring it in for 1 minute.

Add the chopped tomatoes and chicken stock, again stirring gently to incorporate. Bring to the boil, then put a lid on and slide the dish into the oven to bake for 20 minutes.

Take the dish out of the oven and leave to stand with the lid on for 5 minutes. Carefully lift off the lid, stir through the chopped basil and serve up your one-pot wonder.

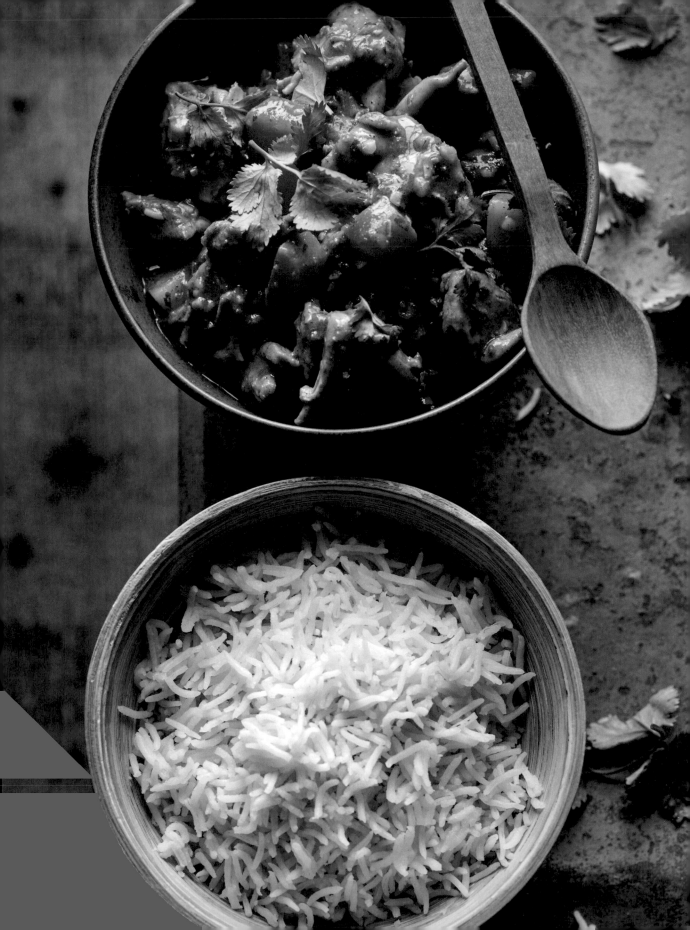

POST-WORKOUT
◆GOOD TO FREEZE

EASY PEASY JAPANESE-Y CURRY

Another curry from another part of the world. I love using different spices and flavours and this one really packs a punch. If you prefer a less spicy version just use half the chilli powder.

◆PREP 10 MINS
◆COOK 25 MINS

1 tbsp coconut oil
5 spring onions, finely sliced
small bunch of coriander, stalks and leaves separated
3 cloves garlic, finely chopped
3cm fresh ginger, finely chopped
1 large potato, peeled and cut into 1.5cm cubes
1 large carrot, cut into 1cm cubes
8 boneless and skinless chicken thighs, cut into 3cm chunks
1 heaped tbsp curry powder
1 tsp mild chilli powder
1 tbsp plain flour
300ml chicken stock
rice, to serve

Melt the coconut oil in a large saucepan over a medium to high heat. When it is hot, add the spring onions. Finely chop the coriander stalks and scrape those in too, followed by the garlic, ginger, potato and carrot. Stir-fry for 2 minutes.

Slide in all of the chopped chicken and fry for a further minute.

Reduce the heat a little, sprinkle in both the curry powder and the chilli powder and continue to fry, stirring almost constantly for 1 minute.

Drop in the flour and continue to stir-fry for a further 30 seconds before pouring in the stock.

Increase the heat and while stirring very regularly, bring the mixture up to the boil. Lower to a simmer and cook for 15 minutes, until the potato and carrots are cooked through, while still holding their shape, and the chicken thigh pieces are fully cooked. Check by slicing into one of the larger pieces to make sure the meat is white all the way through, with no raw pink bits left.

Stir the coriander leaves through the curry and serve with rice.

POST-WORKOUT

STOCKY POTATOES WITH ROAST CHICKEN

This is a real plate of comfort food. It makes a great alternative to a Sunday roast. Cooking the chicken with the skin on makes it nice and crispy while keeping the chicken moist.

➤ PREP 15 MINS
➤ COOK 1 HR 15 MINS

2 tbsp olive oil

2 onions, sliced

3 sprigs of thyme

2 cloves garlic, bashed and left whole

4 potatoes, peeled and thinly sliced (Maris Piper or King Edward are perfect)

salt and pepper

700ml hot chicken stock

8 chicken breasts, skin-on

steamed kale and carrots, to serve

Equipment
35 x 25cm roasting tray

Preheat your oven to 180°C (fan 160°C/gas mark 4).

Heat half of the oil in a frying pan over a medium to high heat. When it is hot, add the onions and cook, stirring regularly for 8 minutes, or until soft and starting to colour. Add the thyme and garlic, reduce the heat to medium and cook for 5 minutes.

Lay half of the sliced potatoes onto the bottom of the large roasting tray. Spoon over the onion and garlic mixture and then lay the remaining spuds on top.

Season generously with salt and pepper, then pour over the hot stock. Roast the potatoes in the oven for 50 minutes without covering, until tender and browning nicely on the top. If you think the potatoes are burning then cover the tray with tin foil.

Meanwhile, heat half of the remaining oil in a large frying pan over a medium to high heat. When it is hot, lay four of the chicken breasts into the pan, skin-side down. Fry for about 4–5 minutes, or until the skin has turned golden and crisp. Flip the chicken and fry for 1 minute on the flesh side, then transfer to a plate and repeat with the remaining oil and chicken breasts.

When the potatoes have been cooking for 50 minutes, remove the tray from the oven and put the chicken breasts directly on top of the spuds, skin-side up. Slide the tray back into the oven and roast for a further 12 minutes, or until the chicken is cooked through. Check by slicing into one of the larger pieces to make sure the meat is white all the way through, with no raw pink bits left.

Remove the tray from the oven and leave the whole lot to rest for 4 minutes before serving the roast potatoes and chicken with the steamed veggies.

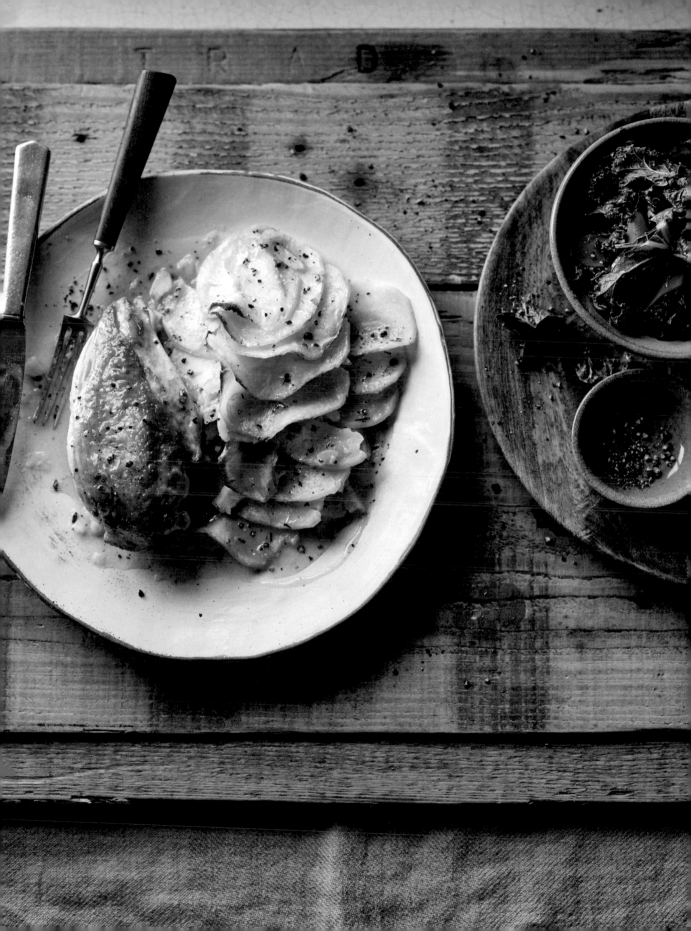

Serves 4

POST-WORKOUT
→**LOW & SLOW**
→**GOOD TO FREEZE**

→**PREP 15 MINS**
→**COOK 2 HRS 30 MINS**

1½ tbsp olive oil

4 large shallots, cut in half lengthways

3 carrots, cut into thirds

3 cloves garlic, bashed and left whole

3 celery sticks, cut into thirds

1.25kg stewing beef, cut into 3cm chunks

1 aubergine, cut into 2cm chunks

1 tbsp tomato puree

1 star anise

1 bay leaf

1 jar of roasted red peppers, drained and roughly chopped

1 litre beef stock

200g chestnut mushrooms, brushed clean and roughly sliced

To serve
large bunch of parsley, roughly chopped
cooked rice

CHUNKY BEEF & VEG STEW

This is a great one for batch cooking and storing in the fridge or freezer for a busy week. Once it's prepped you can sit, relax and come back later to serve it up.

Heat a third of the oil in a large saucepan or hob-proof casserole dish over a medium heat and then add the shallots, carrots, garlic and celery and fry gently for about 5 minutes.

Meanwhile, heat another third of the oil in a large frying pan over a high heat. When it is hot, carefully add half the meat and fry for about 5 minutes, or until dark brown all over. Transfer the browned meat to a plate and repeat the process with the remaining oil and beef.

When the vegetables have been sweating for 5 minutes and are beginning to soften, add the aubergine, tomato puree, star anise and bay leaf to the pan or dish and continue to stir-fry for a further 2 minutes. Slide the browned meat from the plate in along with any juices. Add the red peppers and the beef stock.

Bring to the boil and then reduce to a simmer for 2 hours, topping up with a little extra water if it starts to look dry.

Add the sliced mushrooms and continue to cook for a further 15 minutes, or until the meat is meltingly tender and the mushrooms are cooked through.

Stir through a load of chopped parsley and serve up with a pile of rice.

★ *THE KEY TO ANY STEW IS TO BROWN THE MEAT REALLY WELL: DON'T BE AFRAID TO FRY THE MEAT UNTIL IT IS REALLY DARK BROWN.*

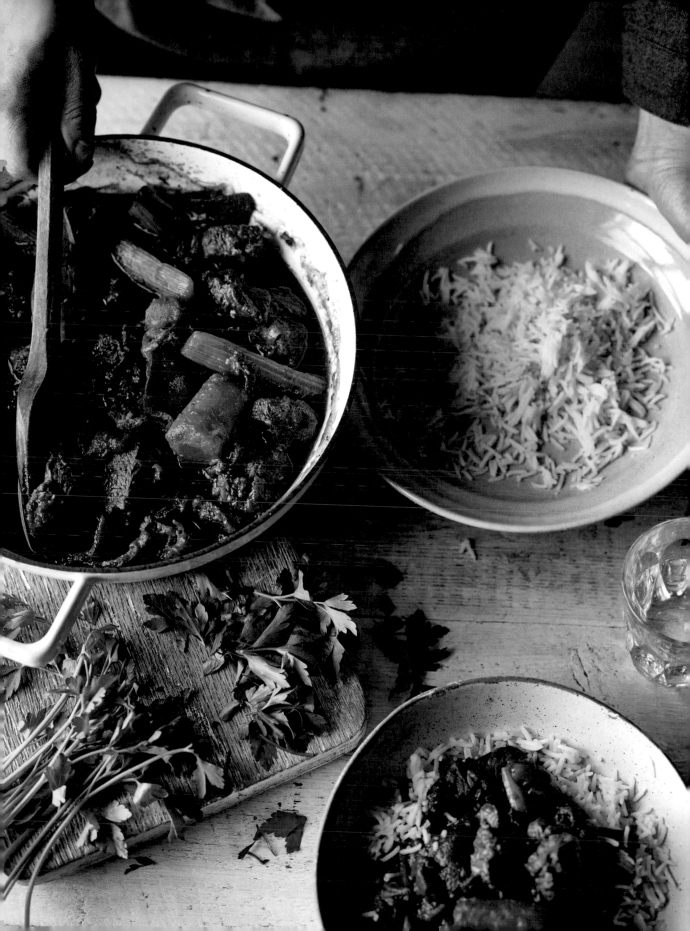

POST-WORKOUT
→BBQ

HONEY-GLAZED CHICKEN THIGHS WITH CUCUMBER & GINGER RICE

This recipe will blow everyone away at your next barbecue. The rice makes the perfect side dish for loads of barbecue classics.

→**PREP 15 MINS,
  PLUS MARINATING TIME**
→**COOK 20 MINS**

1.25kg boneless and skinless chicken thighs

75g light soy sauce

75ml rice wine vinegar

50g runny honey

3 cloves garlic, minced

750g pre-cooked rice

1 cucumber, de-seeded and diced

10 radishes, trimmed and roughly halved

4 spring onions, finely sliced

4cm fresh ginger

2 tsp toasted sesame oil

salt

2 red chillies, de-seeded and finely sliced – optional

green salad, to serve

Place the chicken thighs into a dish and pour over the soy sauce, 25ml of the vinegar and the honey. Dollop in the garlic, give the whole lot a good mix to cover the chicken, and leave to marinate in the fridge for at least 2 hours.

Fire up the barbecue, if using. About 30 minutes before you're ready to cook, remove the chicken from the fridge and allow to rest at room temperature.

Lay the thighs flat over the hot barbecue and cook for 6–8 minutes on each side, until the chicken is fully cooked through. If you're using a griddle pan, cook for about 4 minutes on each side, until the chicken is cooked through. Check by slicing into one of the larger pieces to make sure the meat is white all the way through, with no raw pink bits left. If you're unsure, transfer them to the oven, preheated to 220°C (fan 200°C/gas mark 7), for another 5 minutes.

While the chicken is cooking, zap the rice in the microwave, then tip it into a bowl. Chuck in the prepared cucumber, radishes and spring onions.

Grate the ginger over a clean cloth or muslin and then squeeze the juice into a small bowl. Whisk the remaining rice wine vinegar into the ginger juice along with the sesame oil. Pour the dressing over the rice, season with a good pinch of salt and mix the whole lot together.

By now your chicken should be done, so remove it from the hot barbecue or griddle pan and leave to rest for 5 minutes before topping with the red chillies, if using. Serve the chicken alongside the rice and a small green salad.

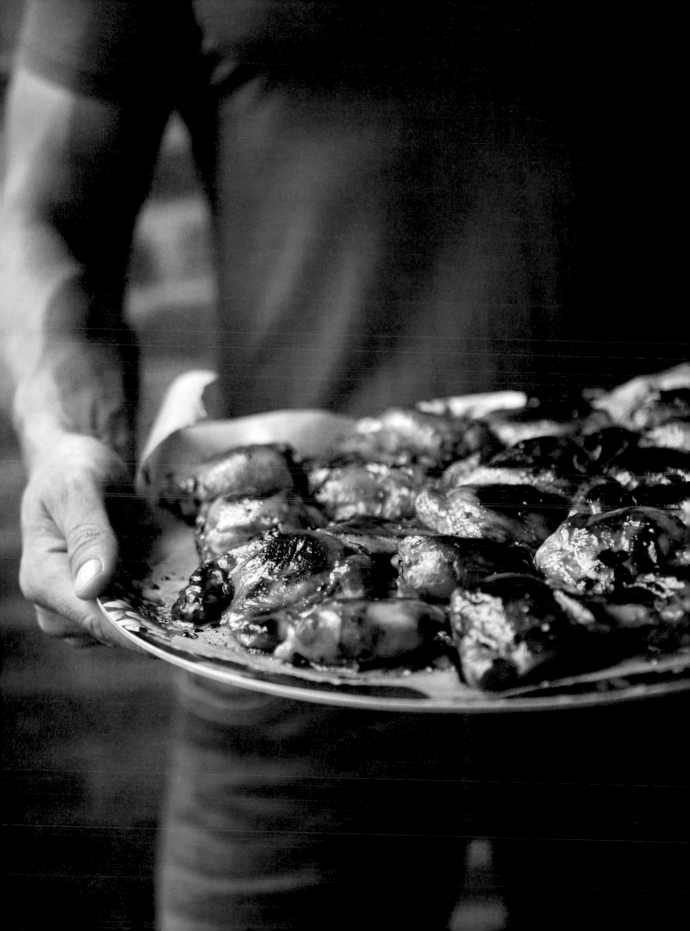

POST-WORKOUT
➡BBQ

TANDOORI CHICKEN WITH CHICKPEA SALAD & CHAPPATTIS

This meal is going to take your barbecue to the next level. The chicken tastes awesome and the homemade chappattis are really easy to make. You'll feel proud when you serve this one to friends.

**➡PREP 15 MINS,
  PLUS MARINATING TIME**
➡COOK 20 MINS

1.25kg boneless and skinless chicken thighs

400g zero-fat yoghurt

1 tsp ground cumin

2 tsp ground paprika

1 tsp ground coriander

2 tsp garam masala

1 tsp ground turmeric

4cm fresh ginger, grated

4 cloves garlic, minced

400g wholemeal flour, plus a little extra for dusting

1 lime, cut into wedges, to serve

Tip the chicken thighs into a large dish. Mix together the yoghurt with the ground spices, ginger and garlic, then pour the whole lot over the chicken pieces. Give them a good stir to coat the chicken and leave to marinate for at least 2 hours.

While the thighs are marinating, make the dough for the chappattis by slowly working 200ml of warm water into the flour with a wooden spoon. When all of the water is roughly incorporated, tip the mixture onto a clean, floured surface and knead it for 5 minutes until you reach a smooth, elastic dough.

Plonk the dough back into a clean bowl, cover with cling film and leave to rest for around 10 minutes.

To make the salad, mix together the chickpeas, red onion slices, coriander, mint, red chillies, cucumber and tomatoes along with the juice of 1 lime. Season, cover and leave to sit at room temperature until you're ready to eat.

Fire up the barbecue, if using. About 30 minutes before you're ready to cook, remove the chicken from the fridge and allow to rest at room temperature.

For the salad

1 x 400g tin of chickpeas, drained and rinsed

1 red onion, finely sliced

1 bunch of fresh coriander, roughly chopped

1 bunch of mint, roughly chopped

2 red chillies, finely sliced – and de-seeded if you don't like it hot

½ cucumber, de-seeded and diced

12 cherry tomatoes, halved

juice of 1 lime

salt and pepper

Lay the thighs flat over the hot barbecue and cook for 6–8 minutes on each side, until the chicken is fully cooked through. If you're using a griddle pan, cook for about 4 minutes on each side, until the chicken is fully cooked. Check by slicing into one of the larger pieces to make sure the meat is white all the way through, with no raw pink bits left. If you're unsure, transfer the chicken to the oven, preheated to 220°C (fan 200°C/gas mark 7), for another 5 minutes.

Take the cooked chicken off the barbecue or griddle pan and leave it to rest.

Divide the dough into either six large pieces or eight smaller ones and roll each into a circle about the thickness of a pound coin on a clean, floured surface. Lay the chappattis directly onto your barbecue or griddle pan and cook them for about 90 seconds on each side. It is more than likely that you will have to cook the chappattis a couple at a time, so just be patient: they don't take long.

When the chappattis are cooked, serve up alongside the chicken, chickpea salad and lime wedges.

SEE PHOTO OVERLEAF ➡

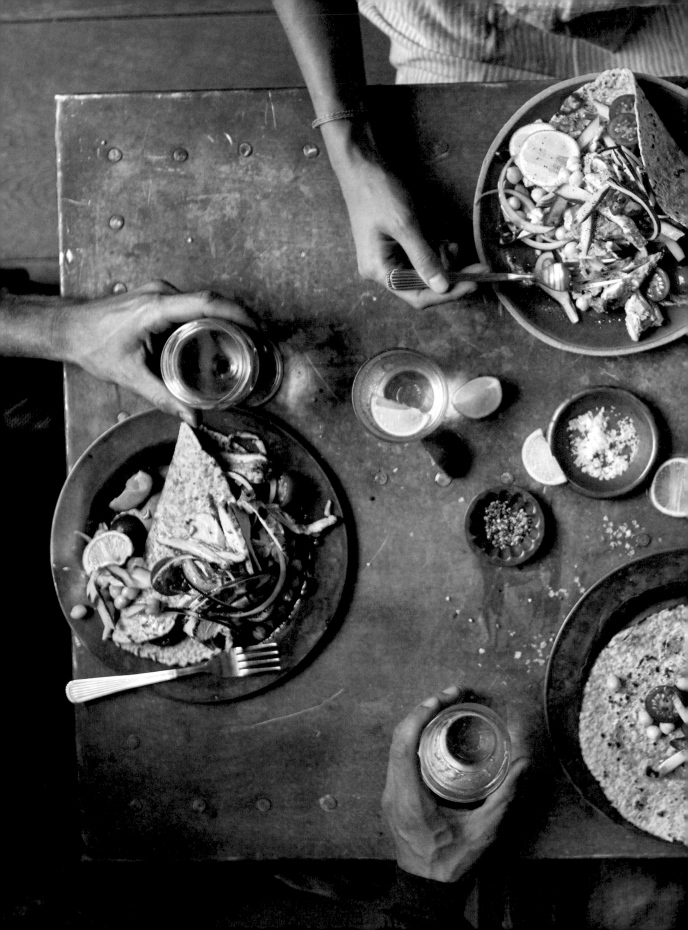

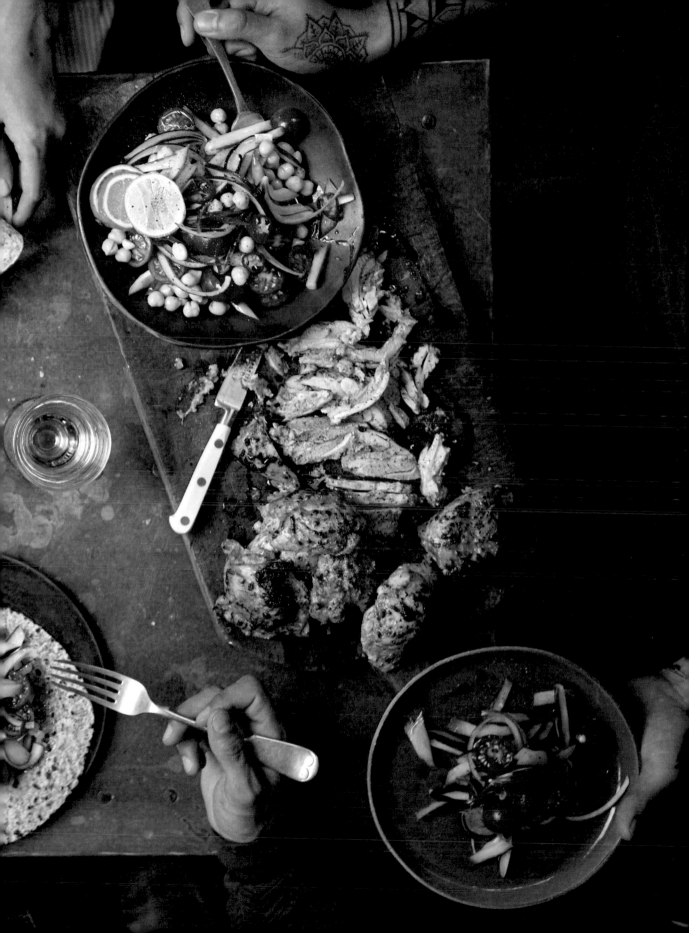

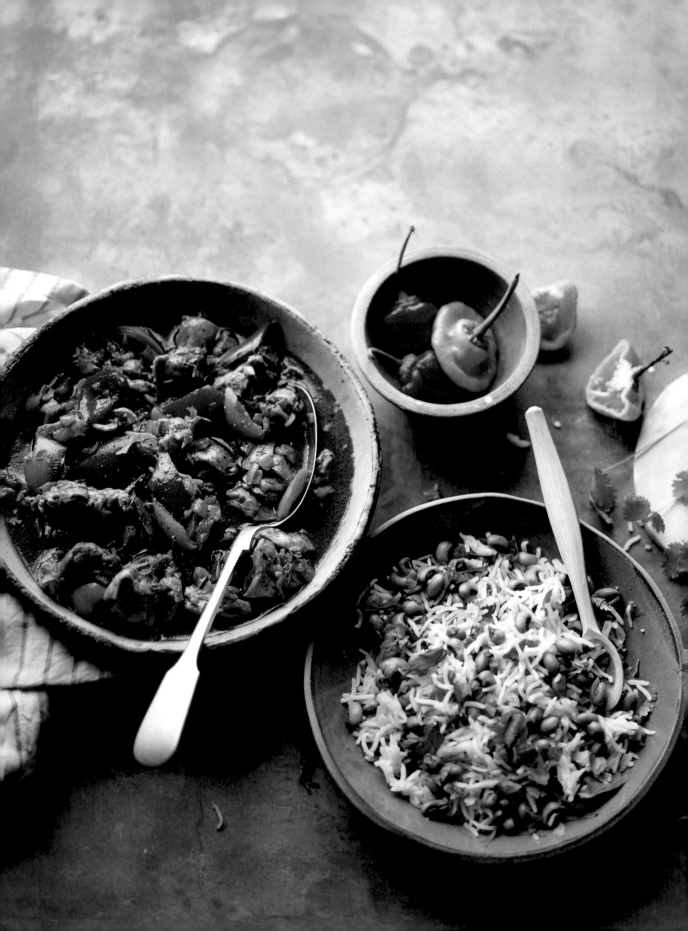

POST-WORKOUT
➧**GOOD TO FREEZE**

CARIBBEAN CURRY WITH RICE & 'PEAS'

Ooh guilty! Another curry. This one tastes authentically Caribbean because it uses scotch bonnet chillies. They are nuclear hot and demand respect, so don't forget to wash your hands after handling them.

➧**PREP 15 MINS**
➧**COOK 35 MINS**

1 tbsp coconut oil

2 red onions, diced

1 red pepper, cut into 2–3cm chunks

1 yellow pepper, cut into 2–3cm chunks

1 green pepper, cut into 2–3cm chunks

10 boneless and skinless chicken thighs, cut into large chunks

4 sprigs of thyme

3 cloves garlic, finely chopped

½–1 scotch bonnet chilli, de-seeded and finely chopped

2½ tsp Caribbean curry powder (I used Dunn's River medium)

1½ tsp ground allspice

1 tbsp tomato puree

200ml chicken stock

400g pre-cooked rice

1 x 400g tin of black eye beans, drained and rinsed

To serve
small bunch of coriander, roughly chopped
½ shredded iceberg lettuce – optional

Melt the oil in a large pan over a medium to high heat. When it is hot, chuck in the red onions and pepper chunks and fry, stirring regularly for 3–4 minutes, or until the vegetables just begin to soften.

Crank up the heat to maximum and add the chicken, thyme, garlic and scotch bonnet chilli. Fry for about 5 minutes, colouring the chicken a little. Sprinkle in the curry powder and allspice and stir-fry for 30 seconds, then squeeze in the tomato puree and continue to stir-fry for a further minute.

Pour in the chicken stock and bring to the boil, then reduce the heat to a simmer and cook for 20–25 minutes or until the chicken is cooked through. Check by slicing into one of the larger pieces to make sure the meat is white all the way through, with no raw pink bits left.

While the chicken is cooking, tip the rice and beans into a bowl and stir together. Cover with cling film and zap in the microwave until heated through.

When the curry is ready, stir through the chopped coriander and serve the whole lot up with a side of crunchy iceberg lettuce, if you fancy it.

POST-WORKOUT
→**LOW & SLOW**
→**GOOD TO FREEZE**

CARMELA'S SPAGHETTI BOLOGNESE

Carmela is my Italian Nan. I asked her to come up with a recipe for this book and this is her all-time favourite. A simple yet classic bolognese: perfect family food.

→**PREP 15 MINS**
→**COOK 1 HR 40 MINS**

3 tbsp olive oil
2 onions, diced
1 large carrot, diced
1 red pepper, diced
2 celery sticks, diced
4 rashers of smoked back bacon, cut into 1cm strips
1 bay leaf
3 cloves garlic, finely chopped
4 sprigs of thyme
2 tbsp tomato puree
1 x 400g tin of chopped tomatoes
300–500ml beef stock
700g reduced-fat beef mince
500g turkey mince

To serve
cooked spaghetti
rocket leaves
grated parmesan

Heat 2 tablespoons of the oil in a very large saucepan over a medium to high heat. When it is hot, add the onions, carrot, red pepper and celery and fry, stirring occasionally for about 8 minutes, or until the vegetables have softened a little.

Add the bacon strips, bay leaf, garlic and thyme to the mixture and continue to fry for another 3 minutes. Squeeze in the tomato puree and mix in. Increase the heat to maximum and fry the whole lot, stirring almost constantly for 2 minutes, then tip in the chopped tomatoes and 300ml of the stock. Bring to the boil and then reduce to a very low simmer.

Place a frying pan onto a second hob over the maximum heat and pour in a drizzle of oil. Add half of the beef mince to the frying pan and don't touch it; let it fry hard for about 1 minute before you then spread it out a little across the base of the pan. The idea here is to brown off a decent amount of the meat – too much prodding and stirring doesn't help! ➡

★ *THIS MAKES A LOAD OF MINCE, SO WHY NOT COOK IT UP EVERY THREE WEEKS AND FREEZE IN BATCHES? #PREPLIKEABOSS*

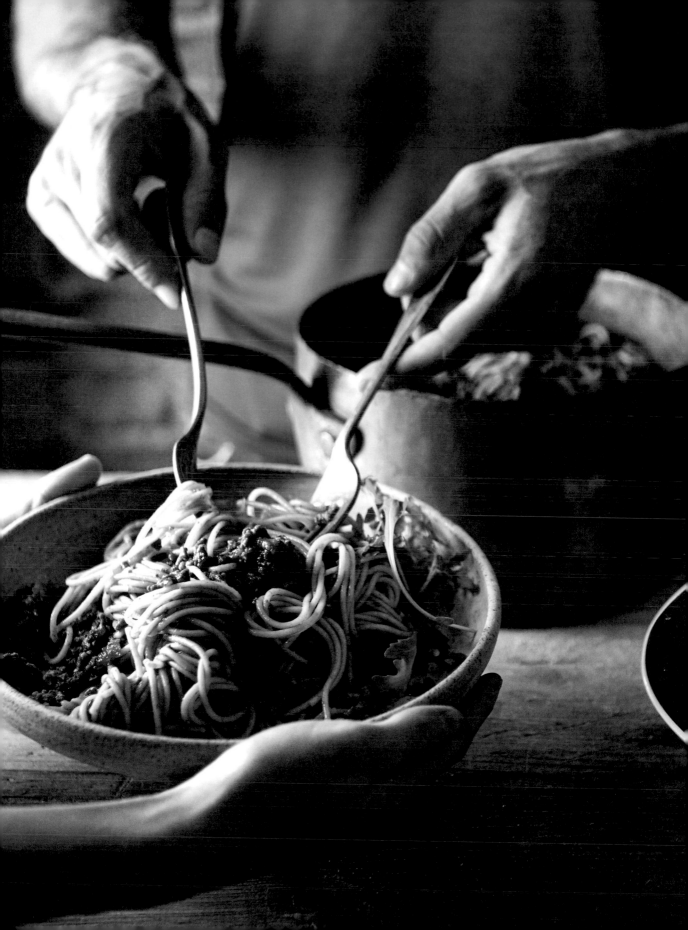

CARMELA'S SPAGHETTI BOLOGNESE (CONTINUED)

Continue to fry the meat until it is all brown, then tip into the lightly simmering tomato sauce. Carefully wipe the pan clean, then place it back over the high heat and repeat the process with a little more oil, the rest of the beef mince and then the turkey mince until all the meat has been fried off and added to the tomato mix.

Increase the heat under the saucepan and bring it to a simmer. Put a cocked lid on top and cook like this, stirring every now and then for 1 hour 30 minutes. Keep an eye on the mince to make sure it doesn't boil dry, and add more stock to the pan if it needs it.

Serve the rich bolognese on top of freshly cooked spaghetti, topped with a little rocket and parmesan.

★ *YOU COULD SMASH THIS BOLOGNESE AFTER 30 MINUTES OF SIMMERING, BUT THE LONGER YOU LEAVE IT ON THE HEAT, THE RICHER THE FLAVOUR WILL BE.*

POST-WORKOUT

CHICKEN SCHNITZEL WITH COUS COUS

Breaded chicken is always a winner and seems to go down a storm on my Instagram page, so here is one of my best.

→ PREP 15 MINS
→ COOK 20 MINS

4 x 150g skinless chicken breasts

300g cous cous or giant cous cous

300ml hot chicken stock

100g plain flour

2 eggs

100g fresh breadcrumbs

1 tsp sweet smoked paprika

a few drizzles of olive oil

½ cucumber, de-seeded and diced

3 tomatoes, roughly chopped into 2cm chunks

½ red onion, diced

½ bunch of chives, finely sliced

½ bunch of parsley, roughly chopped

juice of 1 lemon

drizzle of pomegranate molasses or honey

salt and pepper

Preheat your oven to 180°C (fan 160°C/gas mark 4).

Lay a piece of cling film over a chopping board and place two of the chicken breasts on top. Place a second piece of cling film over the breasts and use a blunt instrument to bash them until they are 1–1.5cm thick. Repeat the process with the remaining two pieces of chicken.

Place the cous cous in a bowl and pour the hot stock over the top. Cover the bowl with cling film and leave to sit while you continue with the recipe.

Tip the flour onto a plate. Crack the eggs into a wide bowl or shallow dish and beat them together. Finally, pour the breadcrumbs onto another plate and mix in the sweet smoked paprika. Take each chicken breast, one at a time, and coat it with flour. Give it a little shake to remove any excess, then dip the breast into the beaten egg and finally lay it into the crumbs, turning it over and patting it to coat as well as possible.

Heat a little oil in a large frying pan over a medium to high heat, and when the oil is hot, lay two of the breadcrumbed chicken breasts into the pan and cook for about 2 minutes on each side, or until they are golden brown. ➡

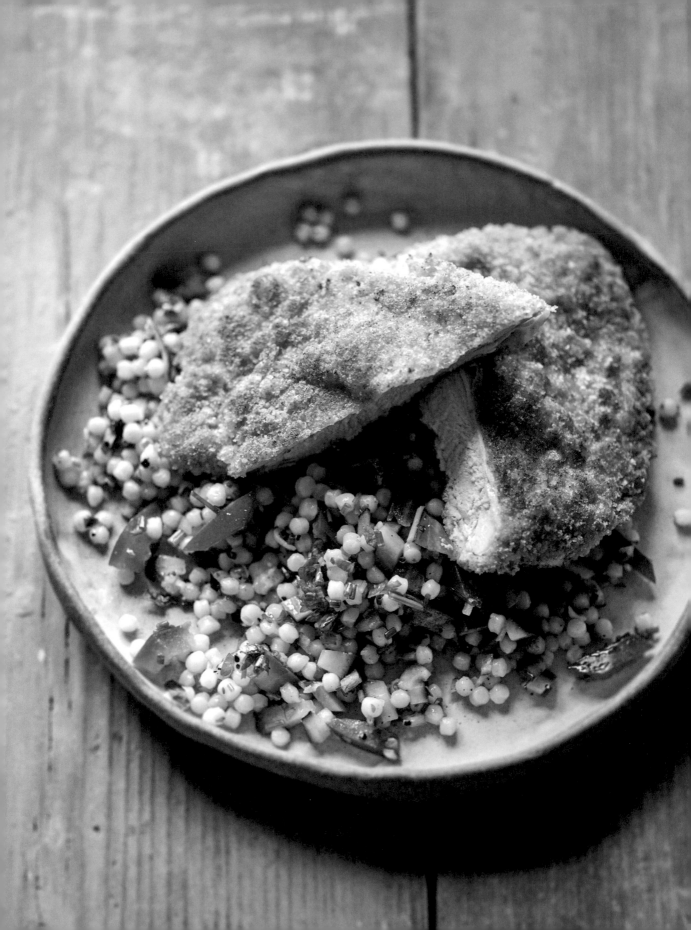

CHICKEN SCHNITZEL
WITH COUS COUS (CONTINUED)

Slide the schnitzels from the pan onto a baking tray, wipe out the pan and repeat the frying process with the other chicken breasts.

Slide the tray into the oven and cook for 8–10 minutes, until the chicken is cooked through. Check by slicing into the thickest part to make sure the meat is white all the way through, with no raw pink bits left.

While the chicken is cooking, use a fork to rake and fluff up the cous cous, then add the remaining ingredients along with a generous pinch of salt and pepper. Give the whole lot a thorough mix.

Serve up the schnitzel and cous cous for a truly tasty meal.

★ *THIS CHICKEN IS JUST AS GOOD THE NEXT DAY – MAKE IT INTO AN ON-THE-GO SARNIE.*

BAD BOY CHILLI CON CARNE

This dish will serve a small army, so throw any leftovers in the freezer and eat later in the week.

POST-WORKOUT
➧**LOW & SLOW**
➧**GOOD TO FREEZE**

➧**PREP 15 MINS**
➧**COOK 2 HRS**

2 tbsp coconut oil

2 onions, diced

2 celery sticks, diced

4 cloves garlic, finely chopped

2 tsp sweet smoked paprika

1–2 tsp cayenne pepper – add more if you like it hot

2 tsp dried oregano

2 tsp ground cumin

1½ tbsp tomato puree

1 tbsp red wine vinegar

50ml Worcestershire sauce

2 x 400g tins of chopped tomatoes

200ml beef stock

1kg reduced-fat beef mince

1kg turkey mince

2 x 400g tins of kidney beans, drained and rinsed

small bunch of coriander, roughly chopped

small bunch of parsley, roughly chopped

rice, to serve

Melt about ½ tablespoon of the coconut oil in a very large hob-proof casserole dish or saucepan over a medium to high heat. When it is hot, add the diced onions and celery and cook for 4 minutes until the vegetables are just beginning to soften. Add the garlic and cook for a further 2 minutes.

Reduce the heat a little and sprinkle in the paprika, cayenne, oregano and cumin and fry, stirring almost constantly for 30 seconds. Squeeze in the tomato puree and again fry while stirring constantly for 30 seconds. Pour in the vinegar and let it bubble down to almost nothing, then pour in the Worcestershire sauce, tinned tomatoes and beef stock. Bring slowly up to the boil.

Meanwhile, melt a little more of the coconut oil in a large frying pan over a high heat. When it is hot, add about a third of the meat (totally fine to mix up the turkey and beef) and fry hard, avoiding the temptation to constantly stir. Fry the meat for about 3 minutes, or until browned all over, then tip the browned meat into the main pot and repeat the process with the remaining oil and mince.

Bring the massive pot of chilli up to a simmer and cook with a cocked lid on top for 1 hour 15 minutes, checking every now and then to make sure your chilli doesn't need a splash more stock to stop it from cooking dry.

Finally, add the kidney beans to the mix and cook for a further 20 minutes, until the meat is lovely and soft and the chilli is nice and thick.

Finish the chilli with the fresh herbs and serve with rice.

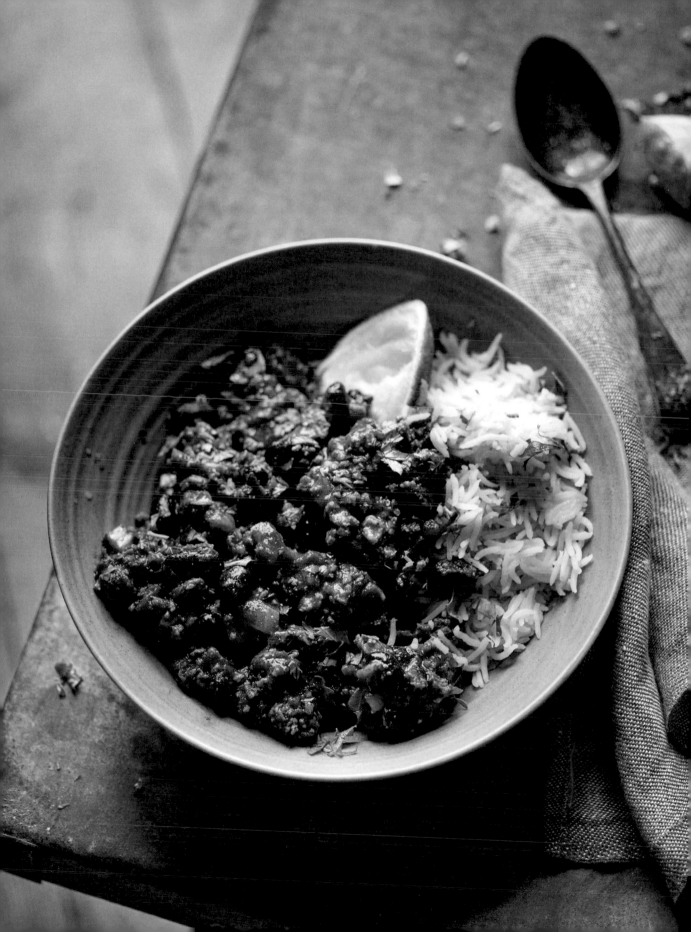

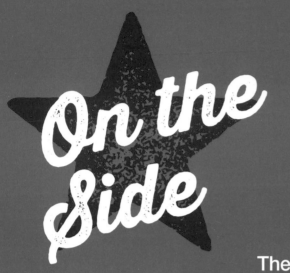

On the Side

These recipes are nice little additions that bring a bit of extra flavour to your meals. They are so quick and easy to make, and you can use them throughout the week.

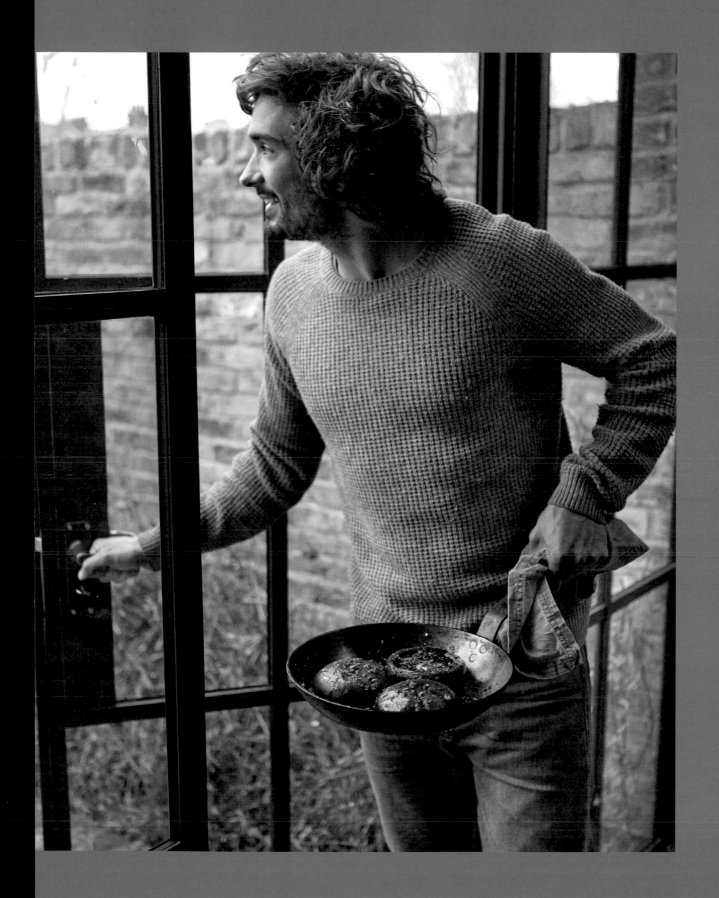

ALL-PURPOSE SUPER SAUCE

REDUCED-CARB
➤GOOD TO FREEZE

I'm a big fan of making my own sauces so I don't have to buy ready-made ones that usually have sugars and nasty stuff added. This is a really simple sauce which you can use on chicken, fish or mince any time of the week. Simply freeze in small containers and either defrost or add directly into the pan.

➤PREP 10 MINS
➤COOK 40 MINS

2 tbsp olive oil
2 red onions, diced
1 courgette, diced
2 cloves garlic, roughly chopped
2 red peppers, diced
1 tbsp tomato puree
1 tbsp balsamic vinegar
800g fresh tomatoes, roughly chopped
20g basil, roughly chopped
2 bay leaves
2 large sprigs of thyme

Equipment
stick or jug blender

Heat the oil in a large saucepan over a medium to high heat. When it is hot, add the diced onions, courgette, garlic and red peppers to the pan. Fry, stirring regularly, for 5 minutes.

Increase the heat to maximum and squeeze in the tomato puree and balsamic vinegar. Fry, stirring almost constantly for 2 minutes, then add the remaining ingredients and 150ml of water.

Bring to the boil and then reduce to a simmer and place a cocked lid on top. Cook for 30 minutes, until the mixture is very soft. Add a splash of water if you think it is becoming dry.

Remove the bay leaves and the sprigs of thyme, then blend the mixture until smooth using a hand-held stick blender or jug blender.

The sauce is fine in the freezer for up to 3 months. If you are planning to freeze it, leave it to cool to room temperature and then portion it out. If you are a family of four, then sealable bags with about 300ml of sauce will work well. If you usually cook for one or two people, then fill up an ice-cube tray and use a couple of blocks at a time.

★ *YOU CAN ADD ALMOST ANY OTHER VEGETABLES TO THE SAUCE AS LONG AS THEY TAKE ROUGHLY THE SAME TIME AS THE OTHER INGREDIENTS TO COOK THROUGH.*

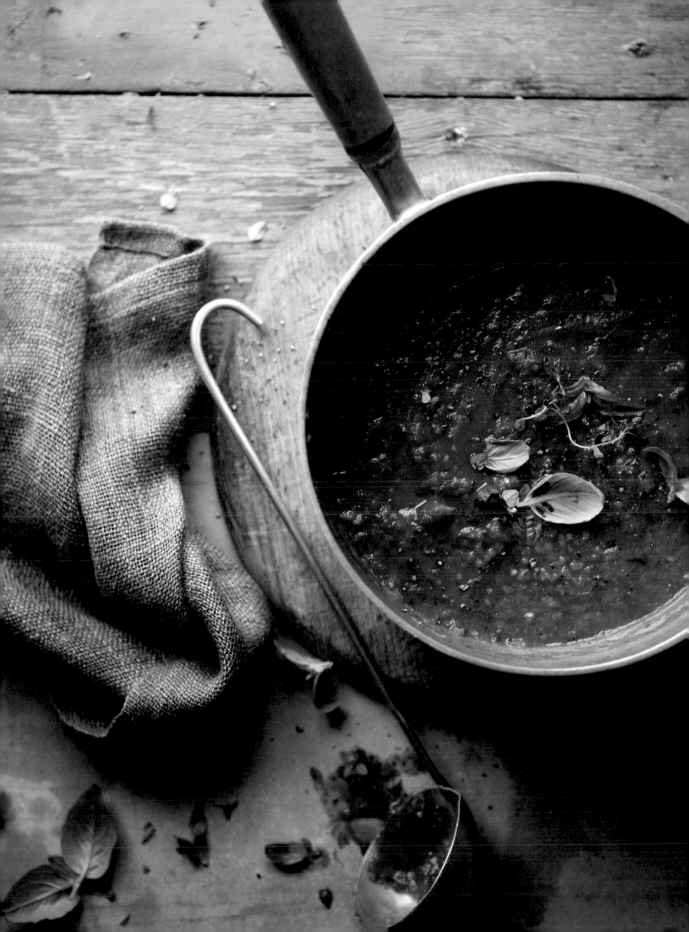

Serves 4

REDUCED-CARB

EASY TOMATO & HERB NO-COOK SAUCE

This sauce tastes amazing alongside steak or tuna. It's really quick and easy to make. Be sure to remove the seed-like flesh part of the tomatoes to avoid getting a watery sauce.

➡ PREP 15 MINS

6 tomatoes

2 large shallots, finely chopped

2½ tbsp red wine vinegar

2 red chillies, de-seeded and finely sliced

bunch of fresh oregano, leaves only, finely chopped (about 25g)

bunch of parsley, leaves only, finely chopped (about 25g)

1½ tbsp olive oil

salt and pepper

Cut each tomato into quarters, and discard the seed-like flesh. Roughly chop the tomato quarters into 1cm pieces.

Scrape the tomato pieces into a bowl and add the remaining ingredients along with a good pinch of salt and pepper.

Give the ingredients a good mix and serve.

Serves 4

REDUCED-CARB

➡**PREP 2 MINS**
➡**COOK 5 MINS**

125ml double cream
salt and pepper
125g blue cheese, roughly broken
into pieces
dash of Worcestershire sauce

BLUE CHEESE SAUCE

There is no easier sauce to make than this one. It's perfect to go with a good steak or some chicken wings. The French blue cheeses are best for this.

Pour the cream into a saucepan, add a little salt and pepper and bring to the boil, then reduce the heat to minimum and start to add the pieces of blue cheese, stirring as you go.

Continue until all the cheese has been incorporated, then take the pan off the heat and stir through the Worcestershire sauce. Serve straight away.

REDUCED-CARB

ROASTED GARLIC MUSHROOMS

These mushrooms are the perfect accompaniment for a steak. I use the big portobello mushrooms but you could use any type of mushrooms you like.

→PREP 5 MINS
→COOK 20 MINS

8 portobello mushrooms, brushed clean

salt and pepper

70g butter, softened

3 cloves garlic, minced

small bunch of parsley, finely chopped

8 sprigs of thyme

Preheat your oven to 190°C (fan 170°C/gas mark 5).

Break the stalk off each of the mushrooms and then lay them gill-side down on a baking tray lined with baking parchment – don't worry if they're a bit squashed together as they shrink during cooking. Season with salt and pepper and roast in the oven for 10 minutes.

While the mushrooms are cooking, beat together the butter, garlic and chopped parsley along with a little more salt and pepper.

After 10 minutes, remove the mushrooms from the oven and flip them over. Dollop a roughly equal amount of the garlic butter onto each of the mushrooms, place a sprig of thyme on top and then roast them for a final 10 minutes.

Remove the mushrooms from the oven and serve.

Serves
4

POST-WORKOUT
→LOW & SLOW
→MAKE AHEAD

→PREP 5 MINS
→COOK 1 HR 15 MINS

24 cherry tomatoes, halved
1 tbsp olive oil
1 tbsp balsamic vinegar
3 sprigs of thyme, leaves only

SLOW-COOKED TOMATOES

These tomatoes become nice and sweet when you cook them low and slow.

Preheat your oven to 140ºC (fan 120°C/gas mark 1).

Place the tomatoes cut-side up on a non-stick baking tray and drizzle with the olive oil and balsamic vinegar.

Sprinkle the thyme leaves over the tomatoes, ensuring that at least a couple of leaves land on each tomato half.

Slide the tray into the oven and bake for 1 hour 15 minutes, then remove from the oven and serve.

★ *IF YOU LIKE YOU CAN MAKE THESE IN BULK, COVER WITH OIL IN A JAR AND KEEP IN A COOL PLACE FOR UP TO A WEEK.*

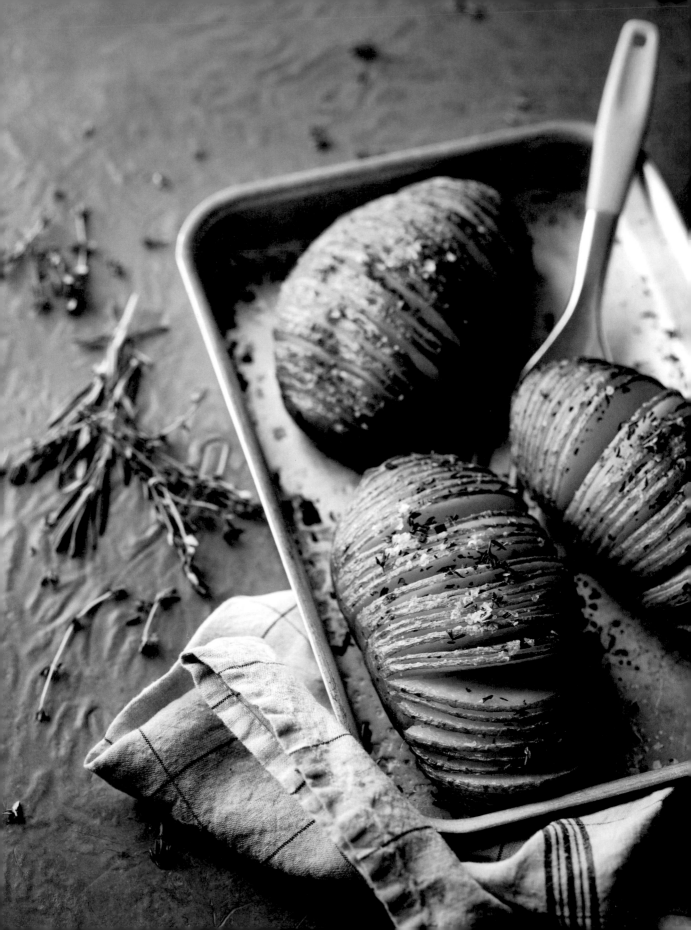

HASSELBACK POTATOES

Check out how incredible these look. I mean, who wouldn't be impressed if you served them up with a nice bit of fish or a big juicy steak?

◆PREP 15 MINS
◆COOK 1 HR

4 large baking potatoes (Maris Piper or King Edward are best)
2 tbsp sunflower oil
salt
4 sprigs of thyme, leaves only
2 sprigs of rosemary, needles only, roughly chopped

Preheat your oven to 190°C (fan 170°C/gas mark 5).

Take each potato in turn and place it on a chopping board. Using a sharp knife, make slits along the spud, each about 3mm apart. Do not cut all the way through to the chopping board – aim for three-quarters of the way through the potato.

Place all the potatoes onto a baking tray.

Use a pastry brush to cover the potatoes with half of the oil, then sprinkle with salt and roast them in the oven for 50 minutes.

Remove the potatoes from the oven, carefully brush with the remaining oil, sprinkle with the thyme and rosemary leaves and then bake for a further 10 minutes, until cooked through the middle and crisp on the outside. Serve.

Starters & Snacks

Here's a few little recipe ideas to kick off a nice meal or impress your friends. Trust me, my Halloumi dippers (see page 196) will go down a treat. My personal favourites are the Egg and chorizo muffins (see page 198) which make an ideal breakfast on the go.

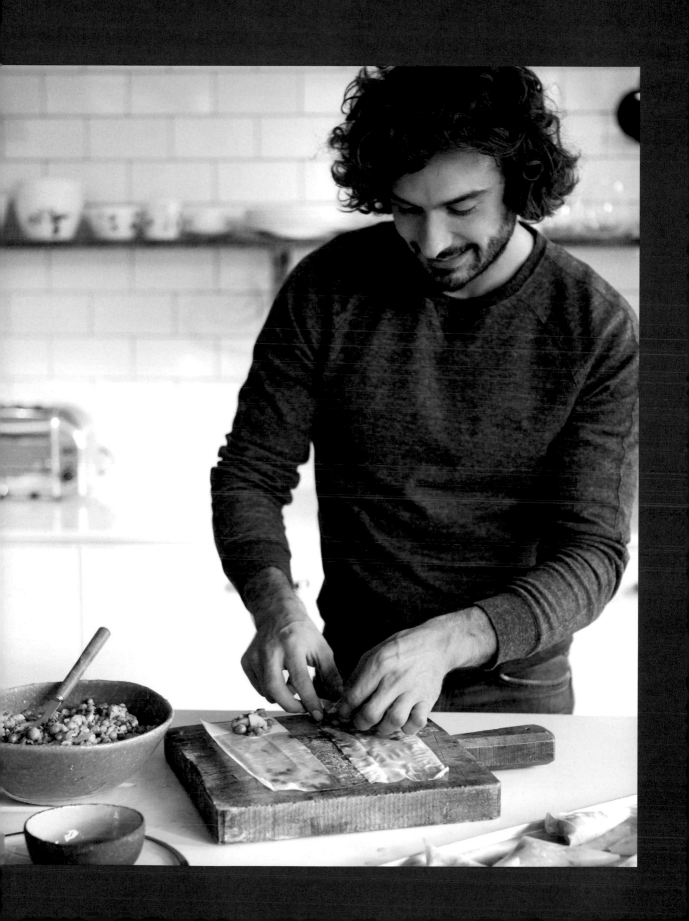

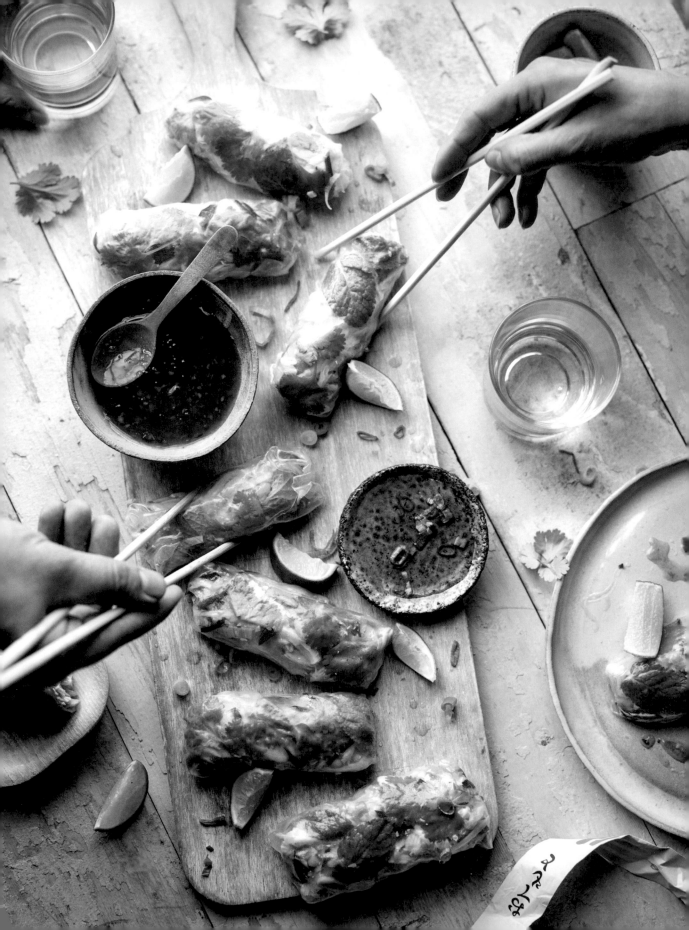

REDUCED-CARB

VIETNAMESE SUMMER ROLLS

If you've ever travelled around Southeast Asia, this recipe will really take you back. With all those flavours of lemongrass, peanuts and sweet chilli sauce, you'll love them. You should be able to buy the rice paper wrappers in large supermarkets.

➜ PREP 15 MINS

250g cooked chicken, shredded

2 spring onions, finely sliced

1 red chilli, finely chopped – and de-seeded if you don't like it hot

2 lemongrass stalks, tender white parts only, finely sliced (about 1½ tbsp)

2 tsp sesame oil

4 tsp fish sauce

1 tbsp lime juice

½ bunch of coriander, leaves only, roughly chopped

½ bunch of mint, leaves only, roughly chopped

½ iceberg lettuce, shredded

40g salted peanuts, finely chopped

salt and pepper

a little olive oil, for greasing

16 rice paper wrappers

sweet chilli sauce, to serve – optional

Put the shredded chicken into a bowl and add all of the remaining ingredients apart from the rice paper wrappers. Give the filling a good mix and add salt and pepper, if needed.

Lightly oil a chopping board and a small tray. Half-fill a wide bowl with warm water from the tap.

Taking one paper wrapper at a time, dip it into the warm water and leave it just long enough to soften – this should be quick, about 5–6 seconds. Carefully transfer the soft wrapper to your chopping board, unfolding where necessary. Place about 2 heaped tablespoons of the filling across the middle of the circle, leaving a gap at either side.

Fold the sides over the filling and then pick up the edge closest to you and fold over the filling. Keep rolling until you fold over the far side where it should stick. Place your completed summer roll onto the greased tray and repeat the process with the remaining paper wrappers and filling.

Serve up the summer rolls just as they are, or with a side of sweet chilli sauce.

Serves 4

REDUCED-CARB
→VEGETARIAN

→PREP 12 MINS
→COOK 10 MINS

2 tbsp coconut oil
2 eggs
75g plain flour
150g panko breadcrumbs
2 tsp nigella seeds
2 x 250g blocks of halloumi,
patted dry and cut into 1cm
slices
300g fresh tomatoes, roughly
chopped into 2cm chunks
juice of 1 lime
½ red onion, finely chopped
1½ tbsp chipotle paste
salt and pepper
1 avocado, de-stoned and cut
into thick wedges
rocket, to serve

HALLOUMI DIPPERS

What did the cheese say when it looked in the mirror? Halloooo me! These make a wicked little snack at a party or barbecue. They wont last long though, so you might want to double up the recipe.

Preheat your oven to 180°C (fan 160°C/gas mark 4).

Spoon the coconut oil onto a baking tray and slide the tray into the oven to heat for 5 minutes while you crumb your halloumi.

Crack the eggs into a bowl and give them a whisk. Tip the flour and breadcrumbs into separate bowls and mix the nigella seeds through the breadcrumbs. Pick up a slice of halloumi and first dip it into the flour, giving it a little shake to remove any excess, then dip into the egg, again giving it a little shake.

Drop the slice into the breadcrumbs and flip around a couple of times to ensure it is evenly coated. Place the crumbed cheese onto a plate and then repeat the process with the remaining slices of cheese.

When you have a neat line of crumbed cheese, carefully slide the hot baking tray out of the oven and lay the cheese slices into the hot oil. Slide the tray back into the oven and cook for 3 minutes, then carefully flip the cheeses over and cook for a further 3 minutes, until the halloumi is warmed through and the breadcrumbs are golden.

While the cheese is baking, mix together the chopped tomatoes, lime juice, red onion and chipotle paste and season with salt and pepper.

Before serving, slide the baked cheese onto a clean piece of kitchen roll and dab off the excess oil. Serve with the avocado, the quick tomato salsa and a big fistful of rocket.

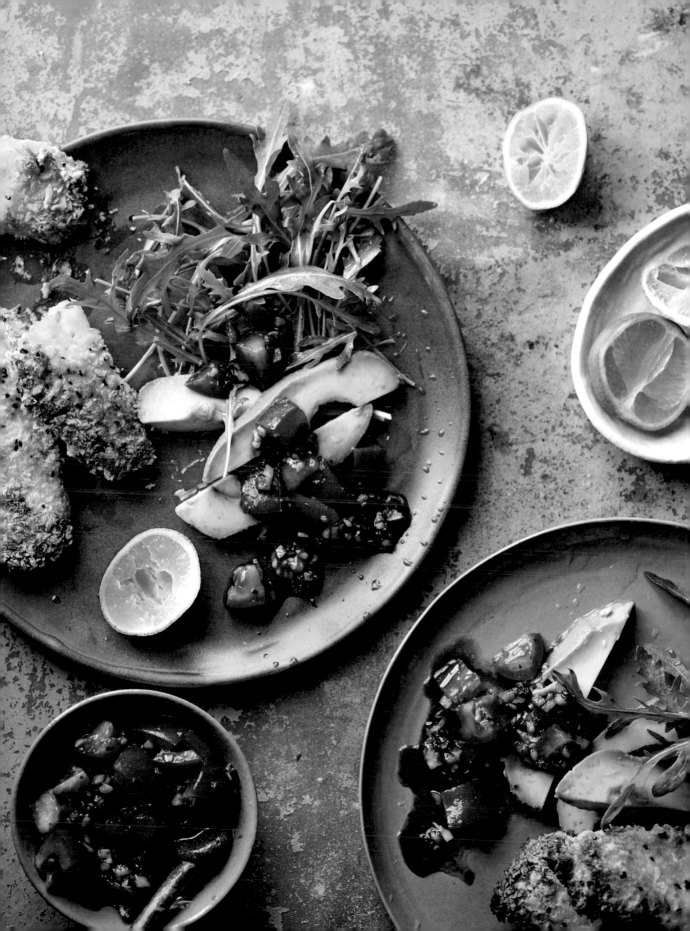

EGG & CHORIZO MUFFINS

These are so easy and fast to make. They include chorizo and cheese too so you know they'll taste awesome. They make a brilliant low-carb breakfast on the go or a snack at lunch.

◆**PREP 10 MINS**
◆**COOK 30 MINS**

½ tbsp coconut oil
120g cooking chorizo, roughly chopped into 1cm pieces
10 eggs
1 courgette, grated
large handful of baby spinach
75g pizza mozzarella, grated
4 spring onions, finely sliced
salt and pepper
a little butter, for greasing

Equipment
12-hole muffin tin

Preheat your oven to 180ºC (fan 160°C/gas mark 4).

Melt the oil in a frying pan over a medium to high heat. When it is hot, add the chorizo and fry, stirring regularly for 3 minutes, or until the chorizo is cooked through. Remove it from the frying pan to a clean piece of kitchen roll to blot off some of the oil.

Crack the eggs into a large bowl and give them a good whisk. Add the grated courgette, spinach, grated mozzarella, sliced spring onions and finally the cooling chorizo. Season with a little salt and pepper and then give the whole lot a good stir.

Grease the muffin tin with the butter and then spoon equal amounts of the egg mixture into ten of the holes, trying to distribute the ingredients as evenly as you can.

Carefully slide the tin into the oven and bake for 25 minutes, or until the muffins are fully cooked through and lightly golden on top.

Don't attempt to take the muffins out of the tin immediately, as they might break up. Give them a few minutes to cool, then get stuck in.

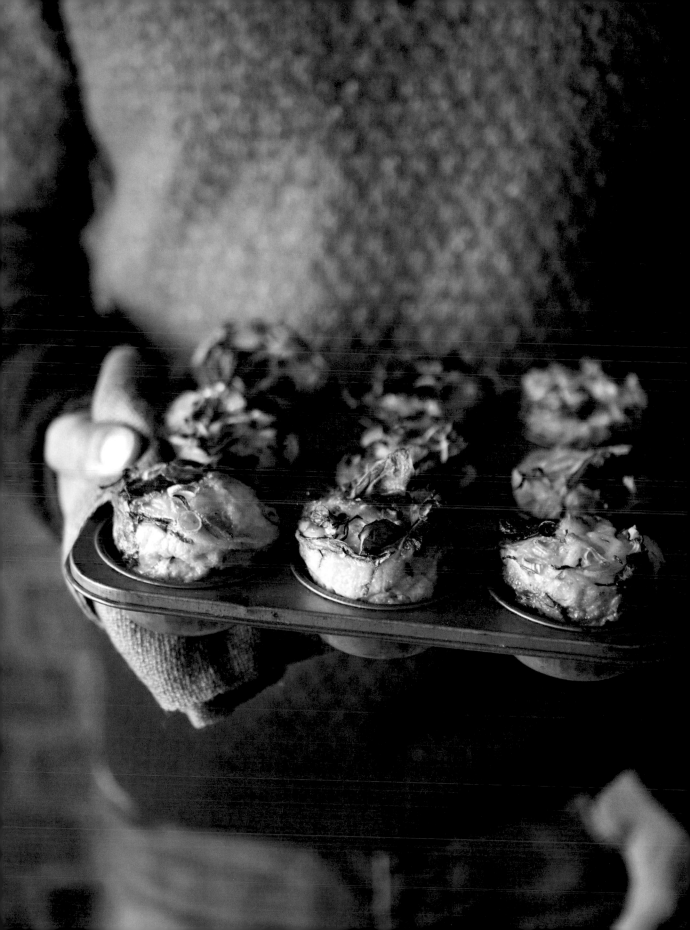

Serves 4

REDUCED-CARB

CHICKEN WINGS WITH BLUE CHEESE SAUCE

If you've got a bunch of friends coming over then this is going to be a real surprise for them. Rather than order a takeaway you can bring the healthy home-cooked version out.

◆PREP 15 MINS
◆COOK 25 MINS

3 tbsp olive oil
¾ tsp sweet smoked paprika
¾ tsp celery salt
black pepper
1.25kg chicken wings
100g soft blue cheese
100g Greek yoghurt
large splash of Worcestershire sauce
celery sticks, to serve

Equipment
food processor

Preheat your oven to 190°C (fan 170°C/gas mark 5).

Pour the oil into a large bowl and add the paprika and celery salt along with a good grind of black pepper. Chuck in the chicken wings and toss them in the mixture until they are as evenly coated as possible.

Slide the coated wings onto a roasting tray and cook them in the oven for 25 minutes, turning halfway through.

While the wings are cooking, place the blue cheese, yoghurt and Worcestershire sauce into a food processor along with a splash of water and blitz until smooth.

Check the chicken wings are fully cooked by slicing into one of the larger pieces to make sure the meat is white all the way through, with no raw pink bits left.

Stack them up on a platter with a load of celery sticks and serve with the tangy blue cheese sauce.

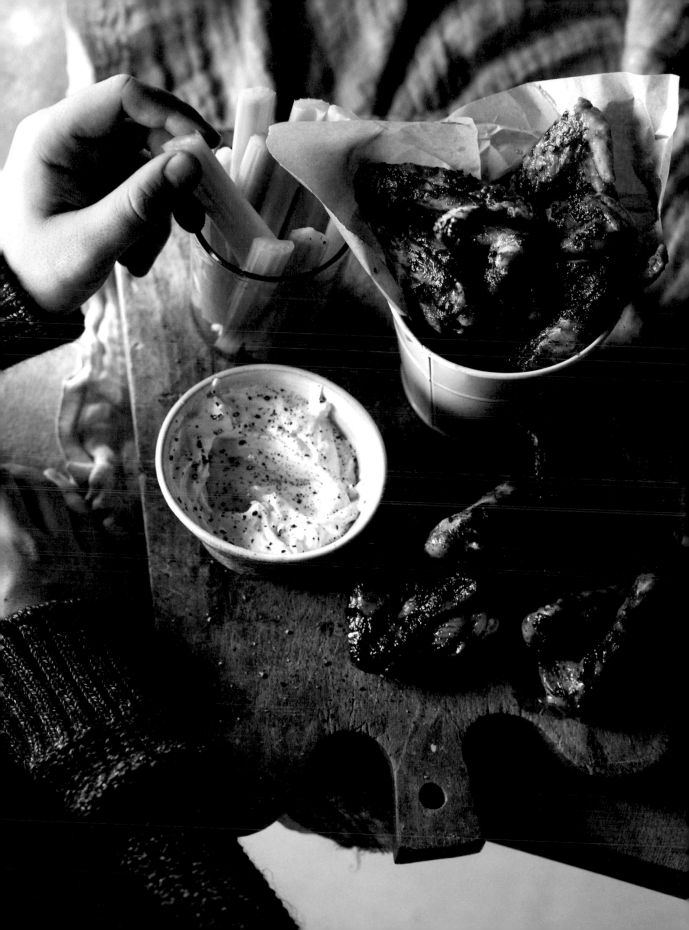

Serves 4

REDUCED-CARB

➡ **PREP 10 MINS,
   PLUS MARINATING TIME**
➡ **COOK 15 MINS**

6 boneless and skinless chicken
thighs, cut into 3cm chunks

2 cloves garlic, minced

3cm fresh ginger, minced

2½ tbsp light soy sauce

oil, for frying

about 100g cornflour

pea shoots and pickled ginger, to
serve – optional

Equipment
thermometer

JAPANESE FRIED CHICKEN

These taste banging. Make these once and you'll be
craving them again and again.

Place the chicken thigh chunks, minced garlic, ginger and soy
sauce in a bowl and mix together. Cover and leave to marinate
in the fridge for a minimum of 1 hour, but preferably anything
from 4 hours to overnight.

Remove the chicken from the fridge about 20 minutes before
you're ready to cook.

Pour oil into a saucepan over a medium heat and, using a
thermometer to check, bring the temperature up to 175°C.
You can also drop a small piece of bread into the oil and allow
10 seconds for it to brown: if it takes longer than this your oil
isn't hot enough, and if it burns, your oil is too hot.

Tip the cornflour onto a large plate or a tray. Take about half of
the marinated chicken and toss it in the flour, then shake off
the excess and carefully lower the pieces into the hot oil. Fry
for 5–6 minutes, until lightly golden and fully cooked. Check
by slicing into one of the larger pieces to make sure the meat
is white all the way through, with no raw pink bits left.

Remove the chicken pieces from the pan and place onto a
clean piece of kitchen roll to drain the excess oil. Repeat the
flouring and frying process with the second load of chicken.

Serve the fried chicken pieces on their own or with pea shoots
and some pickled ginger.

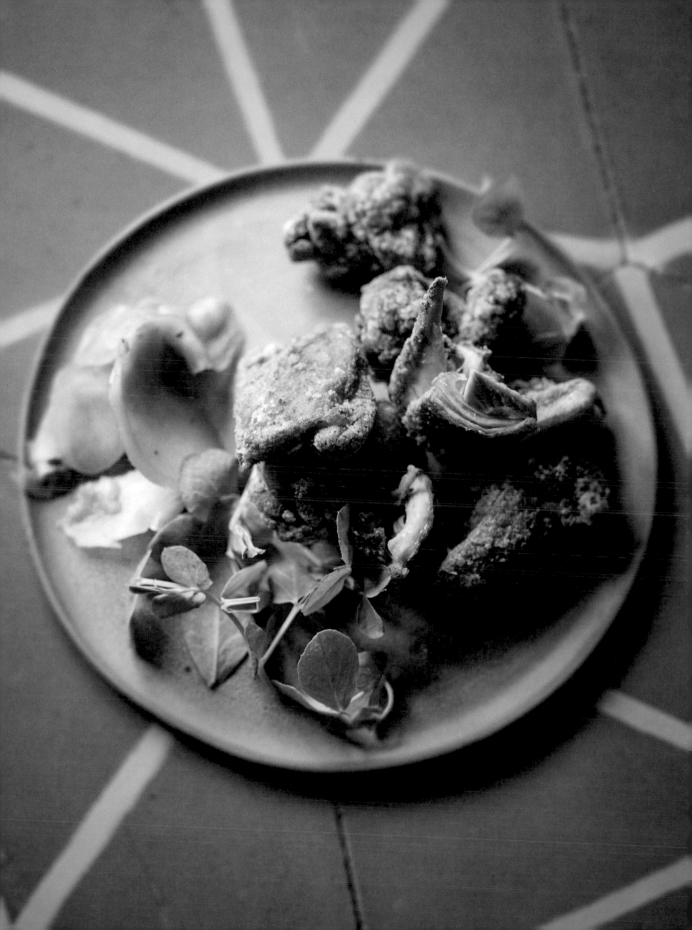

REDUCED-CARB
→ **MAKE AHEAD**
→ **GOOD TO FREEZE**

→ **PREP 15 MINS**
→ **COOK 30 MINS**

3 eggs, beaten

150g fresh breadcrumbs

450g skinless chicken breast, cut into 2cm strips

100ml olive oil

small bunch of mint, leaves only

small bunch of parsley, finely chopped

1 clove garlic, finely chopped

1 tbsp capers, drained and finely chopped

1 tbsp pitted green olives, finely chopped

2 gherkins, drained and finely chopped

juice of ½ lemon

1 tbsp Dijon mustard

salad, to serve

CHICKEN GOUJONS WITH SALSA VERDE

These are the perfect lean snack on the go. You can eat them hot or cold so they are great in a lunch box too. The salsa verde goes so well with them.

Preheat your oven to 190°C (fan 170°C/gas mark 5).

Tip the beaten eggs into a bowl and pour the breadcrumbs into a second one. One at a time, dip each chicken strip into the egg and then roll in the crumbs to coat as well as possible. Lay each crumbed chicken strip onto a baking tray.

Continue until you have two baking trays covered with breadcrumbed chicken.

Drizzle 2 teaspoons of the olive oil over the strips and slide the trays into the oven. Bake for 30 minutes, turning the chicken halfway through the cooking process, until the strips are fully cooked through and crisp. Cut into one of the thicker pieces of chicken to make sure the meat is white all the way through, with no raw pink bits left.

While the chicken is cooking, make the salsa verde by mixing together the remaining ingredients in a bowl until well combined.

Serve up the dippers with your tangy salsa and a big bowl of salad for a seriously good snack.

★ *THESE COOKED GOUJONS FREEZE WELL – YOU CAN EVEN COOK THEM STRAIGHT FROM FROZEN IN AN OVEN PREHEATED TO 190°C (FAN 170°C/GAS MARK 5) FOR 45–50 MINUTES.*

POST-WORKOUT
→**VEGETARIAN**
→**MAKE AHEAD**
→**GOOD TO FREEZE**

→**PREP 15 MINS**
→**COOK 45 MINS**

2 potatoes (Maris Piper or King Edward), peeled and cut roughly into 3cm chunks

2 tbsp coconut oil

1 red onion, thinly sliced

2 cloves garlic, finely sliced

2 tsp cumin seeds

2 tsp mustard seeds

2 tsp garam masala

1 tbsp tomato puree

200g frozen peas

1 x 400g tin of chickpeas, drained and rinsed

1 packet of filo pastry (about 6 small sheets)

PEA, CHICKPEA & POTATO SAMOSAS

I love to make a batch of these and keep them in the fridge. You can reheat them in the oven or just eat them cold.

For the samosa filling, place the potato chunks into a bowl and add about 75ml of boiling water. Cover with cling film, then zap in the microwave for 4 minutes. Leave the potatoes to rest for 2 minutes, then zap for a final 4 minutes. Leave the cooked potato chunks to steam until you need them.

Melt 1 tablespoon of the oil in a large frying pan over a medium to high heat. When it is hot, add the onion and cook, stirring regularly for about 3 minutes, or until just beginning to soften. Add the garlic and cook for a further minute, stirring almost constantly.

Sprinkle in the cumin seeds, mustard seeds and garam masala and fry for 30 seconds before squeezing in the tomato puree and tossing the whole lot together. At this point if you feel the mixture is burning then just pour in a couple of tablespoons of water.

Remove the potatoes from the microwave and carefully peel back the cling film, drain off the water and add the spuds to the pan along with the frozen peas and chickpeas. Toss everything together and stir-fry for 2 minutes, or until you are happy the peas are just warmed through. Leave the samosa mix to cool to room temperature.

When you're ready to cook the samosas, preheat your oven to 180°C (fan 160°C/gas mark 4) and line two baking trays with baking parchment. ➡

PEA, CHICKPEA & POTATO SAMOSAS (CONTINUED)

Melt the remaining coconut oil in a pan. Lay a sheet of filo pastry out in front of you and cut it in half lengthways. Take one strip at a time and brush lightly with some of the melted coconut oil.

Take one tablespoon of the cooled samosa filling and place it in a pile at one end of the strip. Pick up the bottom corner of the filo and fold it over the mixture to create a triangle shape, then fold the triangle shape over itself to seal the gap at the side. Next fold from the top over the filling. Continue to fold the pastry all the way along the strip of filo – by the end of the strip the filling should be completely encased in pastry. By your third samosa I promise you will be enjoying yourself!

Lay the samosas on the lined baking trays and bake in the oven for 25–30 minutes, turning halfway through, until the samosas are golden brown and crisp.

If you want to freeze the samosas, allow them to cool down to room temperature and lay them on a sheet of baking parchment in an airtight container. They will keep for up to 6 months in the freezer.

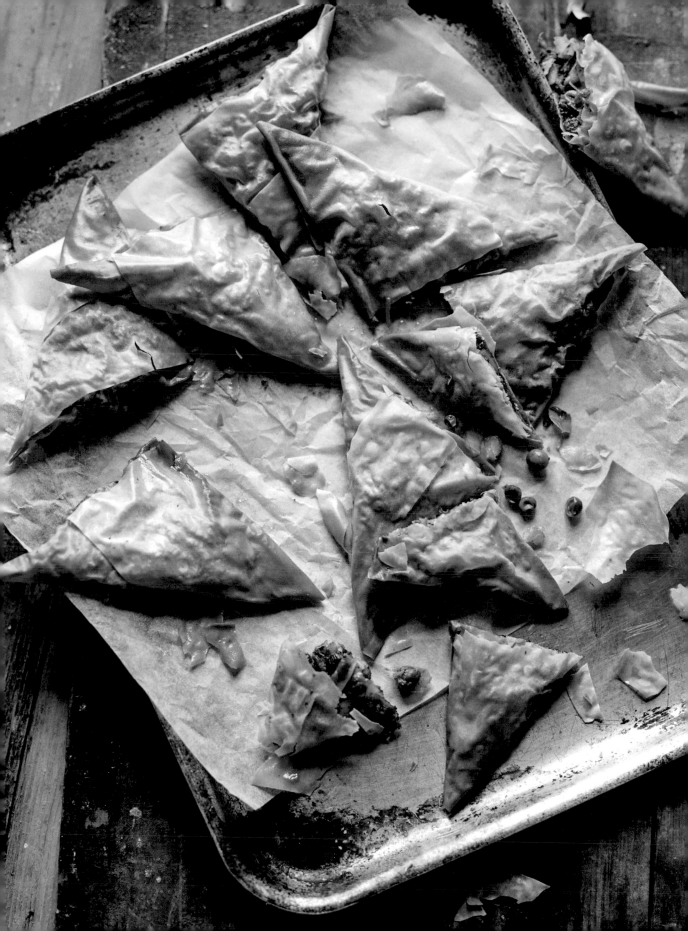

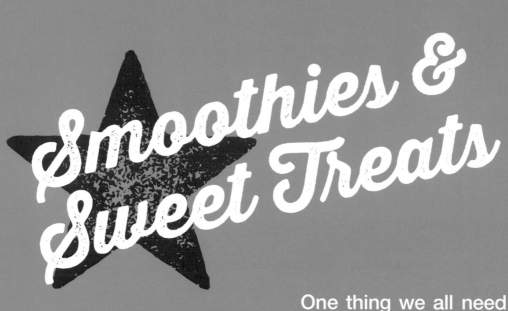

Smoothies & Sweet Treats

One thing we all need now and again is a little treat, especially if we're exercising and eating well most of the time. There are a few healthy ones in here but the naughteee ones really get me going. Roasted maple pineapple (see page 215) may sound a bit strange but trust me it tastes insane. Give it a go! ★

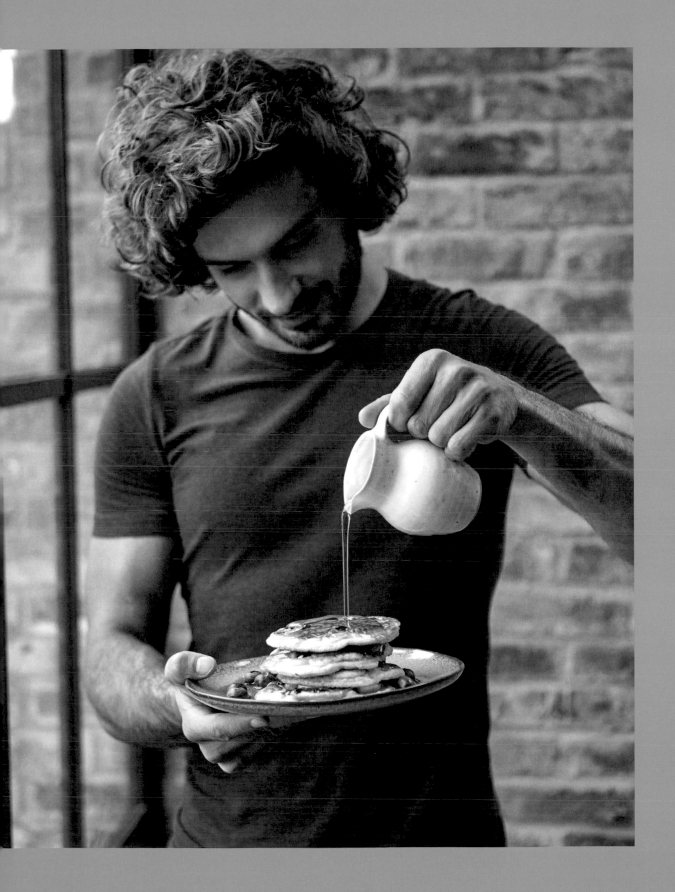

Serves 2

POST-WORKOUT

PURPLE POWER SMOOTHIE

Packed full of antioxidants, this smoothie makes a good snack to have after a workout.

→ PREP 10 MINS

200g cooked beetroot, roughly chopped

1 apple, peeled and roughly chopped

80g frozen raspberries

80g frozen blackberries

500ml coconut water

small bunch of mint, leaves only

Equipment
blender

Place all the ingredients into a blender and blitz until smooth.

★ *MAKE SURE YOU DON'T USE PICKLED BEETROOT!*

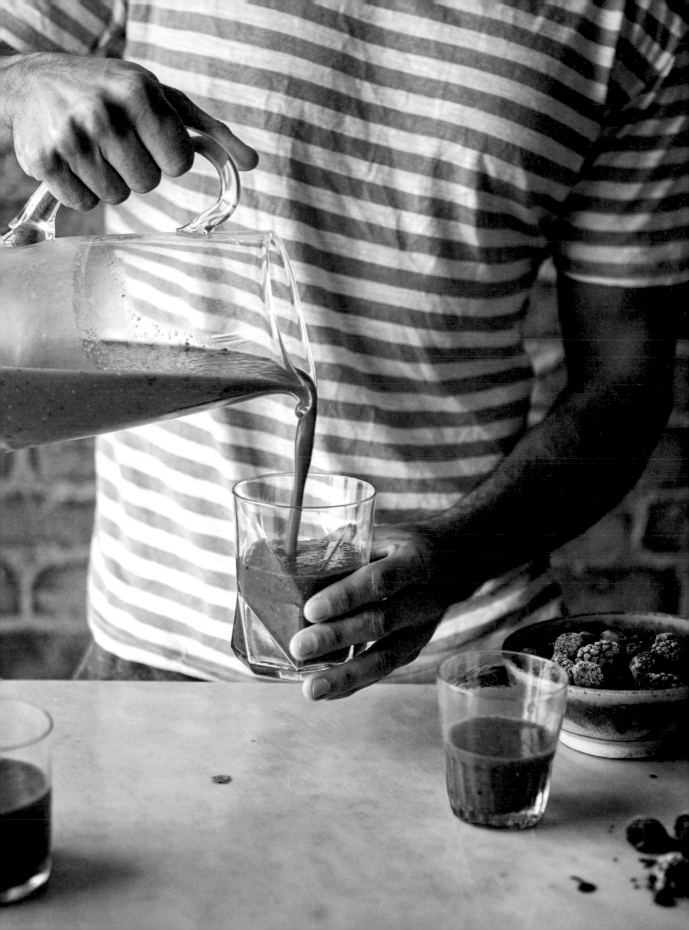

REDUCED-CARB

➡PREP 4 MINS

200ml coconut milk
250ml coconut water
50g desiccated coconut
30g drinking chocolate
50g chocolate protein powder

Equipment
blender

BOUNTY SMOOTHIE

If you like Bounty chocolate bars then you'll love this smoothie.

Place all the ingredients into a blender and blitz until smooth. Drink up!

Serves 2

POST-WORKOUT

BANANA & MAPLE BREAKFAST SMOOTHIE

If you workout in the morning and need a quick option on the go then this is ideal. It contains whey protein and carbohydrates to quickly start repairing damaged muscle.

◆PREP 10 MINS
◆COOK 5 MINS

50g porridge oats
1 banana, peeled and roughly chopped
50g vanilla protein powder
1 large tablespoon malt drink
500ml oat milk
1 tbsp maple syrup

Equipment
blender

Tip the oats into a dry frying pan and place it over a high heat. Heat the oats, stirring them almost continuously for about 5 minutes or until they just begin to toast.

Tip the oats into a blender, add the remaining ingredients and blitz until smooth.

★ *IF YOU LIKE IT FRUITY, ADD A HANDFUL OF BERRIES TO THE MIXTURE.*

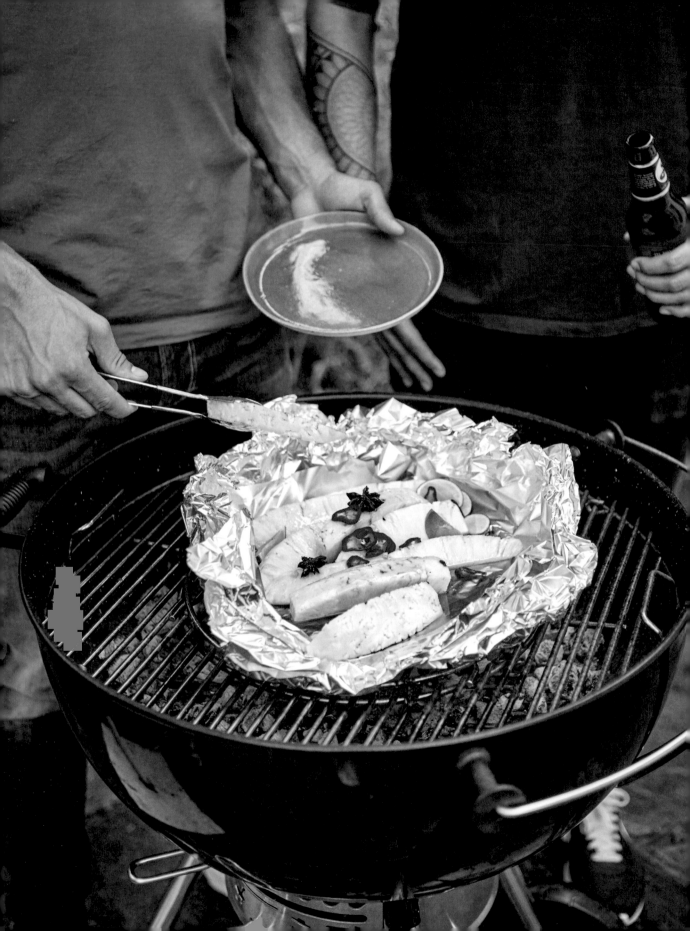

TREAT
→BBQ

→**PREP 10 MINS**
→**COOK 12 MINS**

1 sweet pineapple

2 star anise

2 green cardamom pods,
lightly crushed

40ml maple syrup

1½ tsp vanilla extract

zest and juice of 1 lime

splash of dark rum – optional

1 red chilli, de-seeded and finely
sliced – optional

ROASTED MAPLE PINEAPPLE

This is such an awesome sweet treat to pull out at a
barbecue. Make sure you get a nice ripe pineapple.

Fire up the barbecue.

Top and tail the pineapple using a bread knife. Sit the pineapple
upright on your chopping board and carefully cut the peel
from the sides, using the knife, until you are left with a fully
naked fruit.

Slice the pineapple in half lengthways, cutting out the core if it
is woody. Cut the remaining flesh into twelve long slices.

Spread out a large sheet of tin foil and place the pineapple
pieces in the middle – it doesn't matter if a few sit a little on top
of each other. Place the spices on top of the pineapple, drizzle
over the maple syrup and vanilla extract, and then pull up the
sides of the foil to completely enclose the ingredients.

Lay the parcel on a hot barbecue and roast for 12 minutes.

Carefully remove the package from the barbecue and open
up – be very cautious here as the steam will come shooting
out and may burn. Check if it is cooked by prodding with a
knife – underripe pineapples may need a little longer.

I like to serve mine topped with lime juice and some zest, a
good glug of rum and slices of chilli.

★ *YOU CAN COOK THIS ON A HOT GRIDDLE PAN IF YOU PREFER
– SIMPLY MIX THE INGREDIENTS IN A BOWL AND THEN COOK
THEM DIRECTLY ON THE PAN FOR 12 MINUTES.*

TREAT
→MAKE AHEAD

→PREP 10 MINS
→COOK 40 MINS

120g tahini
100g ground almonds
50g shelled pistachios,
roughly chopped
2 tbsp light brown sugar
1 large egg
about 2 tbsp of sesame seeds
50g melted dark chocolate –
optional

LEANIE TAHINI COOKIES

Everybody loves a cookie right? These quick and easy ones will go down well with a crowd of hungry kids or adults.

Preheat your oven to 170°C (fan 150°C/gas mark 3).

Tip the tahini, ground almonds, chopped pistachios and sugar into a bowl and roughly mix together. Gradually pour in 100ml of boiling water, stirring as you go – the mix will be thick at this point but it's a good workout for the forearms!

When the ingredients are well incorporated, beat in the egg.

Line a couple of baking sheets with baking parchment and dollop on 16 mounds of about 1½ tablespoons of the mixture, leaving a gap between each one.

Sprinkle each mound with a few sesame seeds and then slide your trays into the oven and bake for 20 minutes, or until the cookies have spread and turned golden brown.

Remove the cookies from the oven and leave to cool. If you fancy it, dip half of each cookie into melted dark chocolate, and transfer it chocolate-side up to a piece of parchment paper. Allow to set before serving. Try not to eat the lot yourself!

Serves
4

TREAT

FROZEN BERRIES WITH WHITE CHOCOLATE SAUCE

This is a basic recipe but is the ultimate dessert treat if you have a sweet tooth. Imagine melted white chocolate drizzled over frozen berries. That counts as one of your five-a-day, surely!

◆PREP 5 MINS
◆COOK 5 MINS

300ml double cream
400g white chocolate
25ml limoncello or rum – optional
500g frozen berries
mint leaves, finely sliced, to serve

Pour the double cream into a small saucepan and crack in the white chocolate. Turn the heat on low and stir almost constantly until the chocolate and cream form a smooth sauce. Take the pan off the heat, and stir through the limoncello or rum, if you fancy it.

Scatter the frozen berries in a single layer over a large plate.

Pour the white chocolate sauce all over the berries and finish with the sliced mint leaves. Give the berries a minute to thaw before serving.

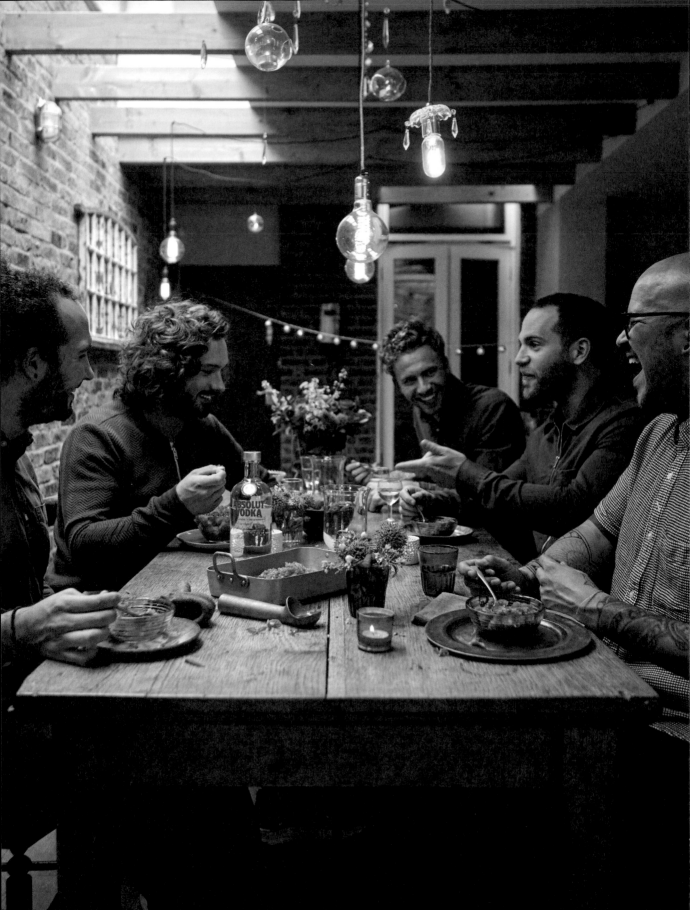

Serves
6-8

TREAT
MAKE AHEAD

**PREP 10 MINS,
PLUS FREEZING**

flesh of 1 small watermelon
(about 800g)
large bunch of mint, leaves
roughly chopped, plus a little
extra to garnish
150g caster sugar
ice-cold vodka – optional

Equipment
blender

WATERMELON & MINT GRANITA

This is so refreshing on a hot day. It's like a posh slush puppy. If you want to make it boozy for adults, add some ice-cold vodka!

Roughly chop the watermelon flesh and place into a blender with the mint leaves and sugar. Blitz the ingredients until they become smooth. You may need to shake your blender about to get really smooth results.

Pass the mixture through a sieve into an airtight container, cover and place in the freezer.

After about 90 minutes, the liquid should just be beginning to freeze around the edges. Using a fork, scrape the frozen sides into the main mixture and stir the whole lot. Slide the mixture back into the freezer.

From now on it's worth checking the mix every hour, and as it becomes solid, scrape the crystals up with a fork and then replace in the freezer. Gradually there will be more ice crystals than liquid and eventually you should end up with a box full of deliciously red ice crystals that resemble a slush puppy.

Serve the granita up as it is, or the way I like it: with frozen vodka drizzled over the top.

TREAT
→ MAKE AHEAD

→ PREP 5 MINS,
   PLUS FREEZING

200g fresh raspberries
1 x 300g tin of peaches, drained
½ banana, peeled and roughly
chopped

Equipment
blender
6-hole lolly mould

PEACH MELBA LOLLIES

These are so easy to make and kids and adults will
love them.

Place all of the ingredients into a blender and blitz until smooth.
Divide the mixture between the holes in the lolly mould and
then place in the freezer for at least 4 hours, until solid.

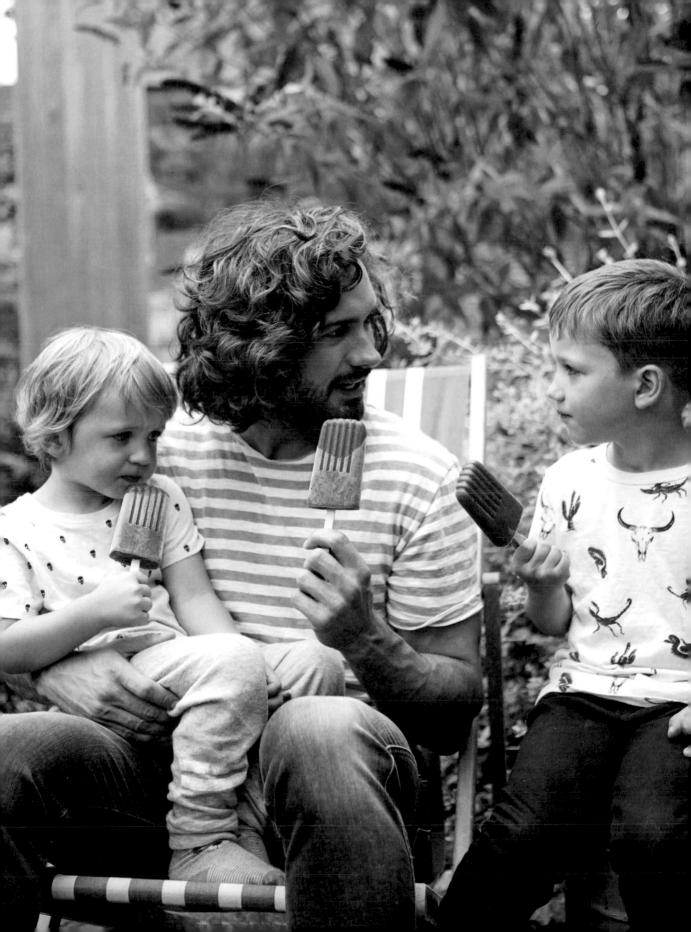

TREAT
◆MAKE AHEAD

◆PREP 8 MINS
◆COOK 25 MINS

2 tbsp coconut oil
100g golden syrup
1 tbsp dark brown sugar
zest and juice of 1 lemon
400g rolled oats
½ tsp ground cinnamon
½ tsp ground ginger
200g raisins

Equipment
20 x 25cm baking tray

CINNAMON & GINGER FLAPJACKS

It's nice to make your own treats at home. If you have a sweet tooth, I think you'll love these easy flapjacks.

Preheat your oven to 170°C (fan 150°C/gas mark 3).

Put the coconut oil, golden syrup, sugar, lemon zest and juice into a small pan over a low heat and stir until they come together.

Tip the remaining ingredients into a bowl and pour the golden syrup mixture over the top, mixing everything together well with a wooden spoon.

Line the baking tray with baking parchment and spread the mixture over the base. Lay a second piece of parchment over the top and then cover the flapjacks with tin foil and bake for 15 minutes.

Remove the tin foil and parchment from the top and bake for a further 10 minutes. Remove from the oven and leave to cool before chopping up into thick chunks and tucking in.

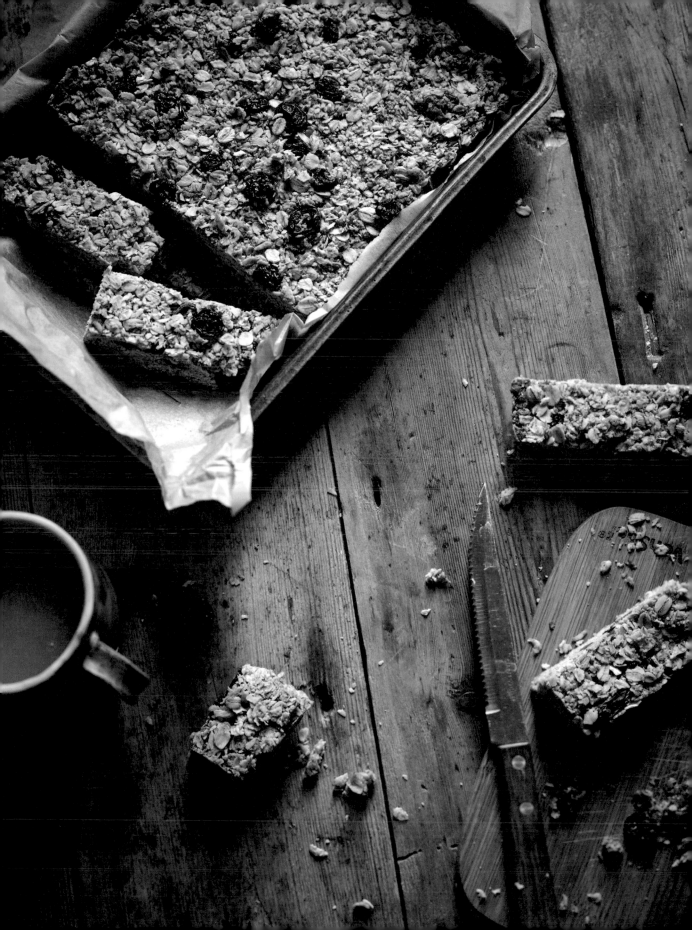

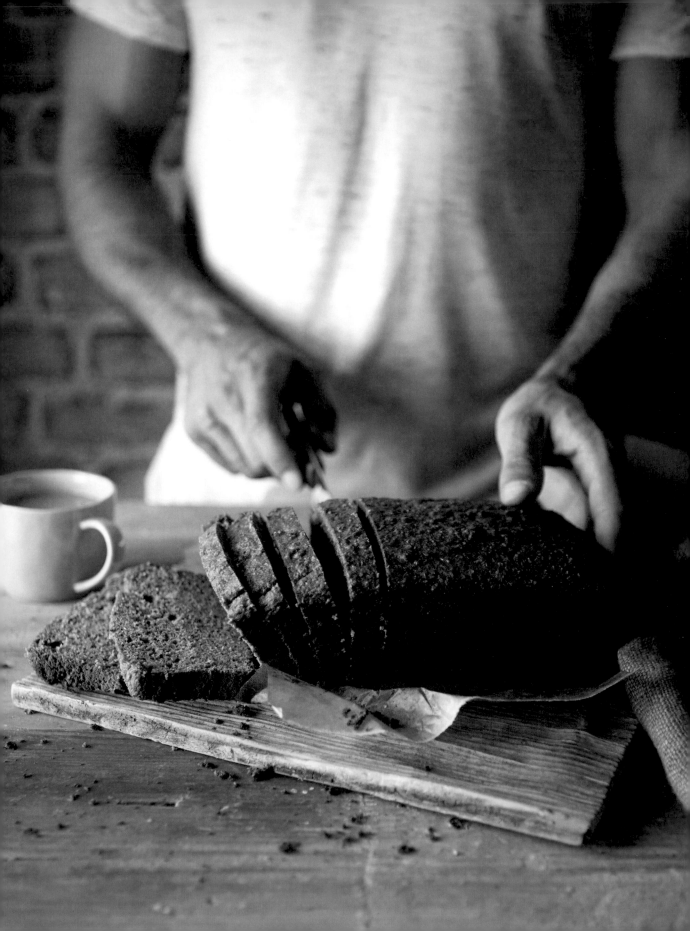

Serves
6

TREAT
→MAKE AHEAD

→**PREP 15 MINS**
→**COOK 1 HR**

150g pitted dates, roughly
chopped into small pieces
75g butter, cubed
25g light brown soft sugar
3 bananas, peeled and roughly
chopped (about 250g)
3 eggs
200g strong wholemeal flour
2 tsp baking powder
¼ tsp bicarbonate of soda

Equipment
1.5 litre loaf tin
food processor

BANANA & DATE CAKE

The key to a tasty banana cake is using over-ripe bananas – the darker the better. This makes a great snack for work or in kid's lunch boxes.

Preheat your oven to 180°C (fan 160°C/gas mark 4) and line the loaf tin with baking parchment.

Put the chopped dates, butter, sugar and 75ml of boiling water into a heatproof bowl, give the ingredients a little stir and leave them to soak and melt for 5 minutes.

Tip the contents of the bowl into the food processor and add the banana chunks and eggs. Blitz until the whole lot is smooth and then tip the mixture into a medium mixing bowl.

Sift the flour, baking powder and bicarbonate of soda Into the mixture, giving it a good beating with a wooden spoon until well combined. Pour the batter into the loaf tin and bake the cake for 1 hour in the oven.

Remove the loaf tin from the oven and leave it to sit for 10 minutes before turning out and cutting up.

TREAT
→ MAKE AHEAD

BANANA, RUM & RAISIN 'ICE CREAM'

Here's a naughty little treat for you to try. It's not double boozy but feel free to add a bit more rum when no one is looking. I won't tell anyone.

→ **PREP 5 MINS, PLUS FREEZING TIME**

8 bananas, peeled and roughly chopped into 3–4cm chunks
60ml rum
60g raisins
seeds of 1 vanilla pod

Equipment
food processor

Lay the banana chunks onto a baking tray and freeze overnight.

Warm the rum up a little in a small saucepan, then add the raisins and leave to soak and cool down to room temperature. You can also leave these to soak overnight.

Slide the banana pieces into a food processor and add the vanilla seeds. Blitz until smooth, then tip the ice cream into a bowl and stir through the soaked raisins and rum from the bottom of the bowl.

Put the ice cream back in the freezer for 30 minutes, or until it has firmed up again, and then serve.

APPLE STRUDEL PIE

This is classic dessert that will go down a treat after any dinner, party or barbecue. It's easy to make but will really impress your guests.

⇒PREP 20 MINS
⇒COOK 45 MINS

750g cooking apples, peeled, cored and cut into large chunks (peeled weight)
90g soft light brown sugar
1 tsp ground mixed spice
½ tsp ground cinnamon
50g rolled oats
175g blackberries
2–3 filo pastry sheets
1 tbsp coconut oil, melted

Equipment
20 x 20cm square baking dish

Preheat the oven to 180ºC (fan 160°C/gas mark 4).

Put the apple into a bowl, add a splash of water, cover with cling film and zap in the microwave for 90 seconds – the idea here is not to cook the apple, but to give it a little headstart before going into the oven.

Tip the apple into a large clean bowl and add the sugar, mixed spice, cinnamon and oats. Give the whole lot a good mix and then tumble in the blackberries and gently toss to combine. Transfer the mixture to the baking dish.

Take a sheet of filo and tear it in half, then scrunch both pieces up and place on top of the fruit filling. Continue with the other filo slices until you have totally covered the fruit – don't worry about neatness or overlapping; there is almost no right or wrong way to do this bit.

Brush the top of the filo with the melted coconut oil, then slide the dish into the oven and bake for 40 minutes. Keep an eye on the pie – if you think it is burning, just cover with a little tin foil and continue to cook.

Serve up and enjoy.

Serves 4

NAUGHTEEE TREAT

GUILTEEE CHOCOLATE FONDANT

My philosophy is, if you're going to treat yourself, at least do it properly. This is the tastiest treat in the whole book if you ask me. Is it lean? Erm no, quite the opposite, but that's why I love it and enjoy it so much as a treat once in a while.

→ **PREP 10 MINS**
→ **COOK 16 MINS**

125g dark chocolate
125g butter, roughly cubed
3 eggs
125g caster sugar
50g flour
4 Lindt Lindor Milk Truffles (the red ones) or Ferrero Rochers
ice cream, to serve

Equipment
electric beaters – optional
4 ramekins

Preheat your oven to 200°C (fan 180°C/gas mark 6).

Crack the chocolate and butter into a heatproof bowl. Place the bowl over a pan of boiling water, making sure the base of the bowl doesn't touch the water. Leave the ingredients to melt, stirring only when they are almost completely melted. Remove the bowl from the pan and leave to cool a little.

While the chocolate is melting, crack the eggs into a bowl and tip in the sugar. Beat together for about 5 minutes (or 3 minutes with electric beaters) until the mixture has increased in volume, is a pale yellow colour and is slightly mousse-like.

When you are happy with the consistency, stir the egg mixture through the chocolate mixture and then finally fold in the flour.

Place four ramekins onto a baking tray and pour equal amounts of the mixture into each one, then poke a Lindt truffle or Ferrero Rocher into the centre of each ramekin – don't worry if the chocolate isn't totally immersed in the batter; the cake mixture will rise over the top.

Slide the tray into the oven and bake for 16 minutes, then remove and leave the puddings to sit for 2 minutes before turning them out, scooping on a big dollop of ice cream and getting stuck in.

★ *YOU CAN ALSO COOK THESE IN DARIOLE MOULDS AND THEN TURN THEM OUT – IF YOU DO THEN KNOCK 1 MINUTE OFF THE COOKING TIME.*

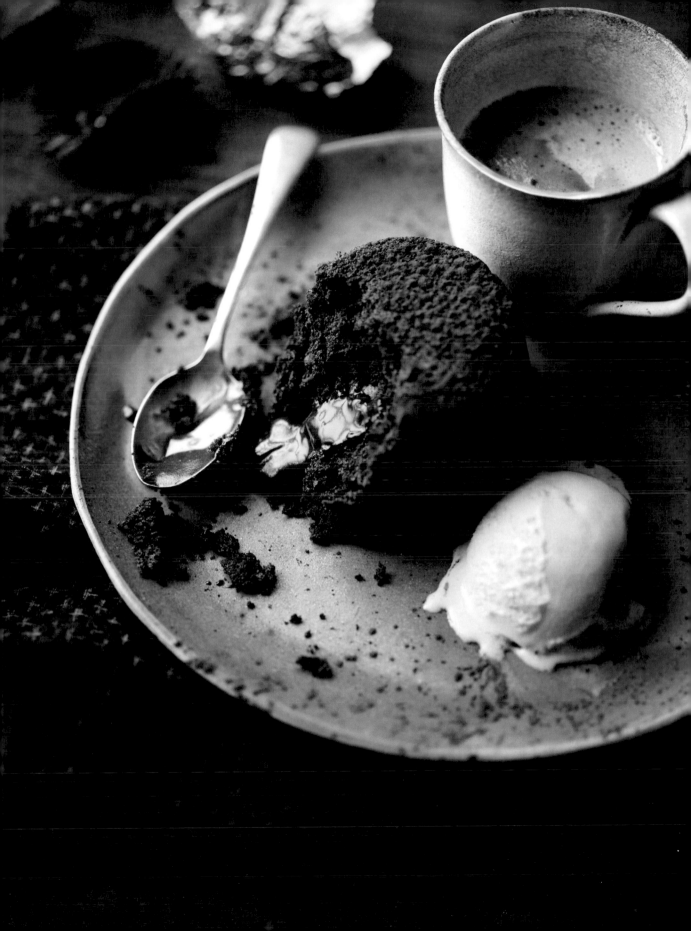

NAUGHTEEE TREAT

STICKY TOFFEE PUDDING

When I see a chocolate fondant and a sticky toffee pudding on the same menu I seriously struggle to choose between the two. This is one of my all-time favourite pub desserts. It legit tastes like a proper pub-made one, too.

→ **PREP 15 MINS,**
   PLUS SOAKING TIME
→ **COOK 45 MINS**

200g pitted dates
190g butter, roughly cubed
100g golden caster sugar
3 eggs
30g black treacle
1 tsp bicarbonate of soda
200g self-raising flour
120g soft light brown sugar
200ml double cream
ice cream, to serve – optional

Equipment
22 x 15cm baking dish
food processor

Place the dates into a large bowl, pour over 175ml of boiling water and leave to stand for a minimum of 30 minutes (you might find that if you have very dry dates they benefit from a further 15 minutes).

Preheat your oven to 180°C (fan 160°C/gas mark 4) and line the baking dish with baking parchment.

Place the dates and all of the soaking liquid into a food processor. Add 100g of the butter, the golden caster sugar, eggs and treacle. Blitz until pretty much smooth – don't worry if it looks as if the butter and eggs are splitting; it will all come good.

Add the bicarbonate of soda and self-raising flour and blitz until you reach a smooth consistency. Tip the batter into the lined baking dish. Spread the batter out so it is fairly even and then slide into the oven and bake for 45 minutes.

Place the remaining 90g of butter into a saucepan with the soft light brown sugar and double cream, and bring slowly to the boil while stirring regularly. Boil the sauce for 1 minute, then remove from the heat.

When the cake is fully cooked, remove it from the oven and prick it all over with a fork. Pour over about 4 tablespoons of the sauce and spread it over the top of the cake. Let the cake stand for 5 minutes, then remove from the dish, cut into squares and serve up with the remaining toffee sauce and ice cream, if you really want to push the boat out.

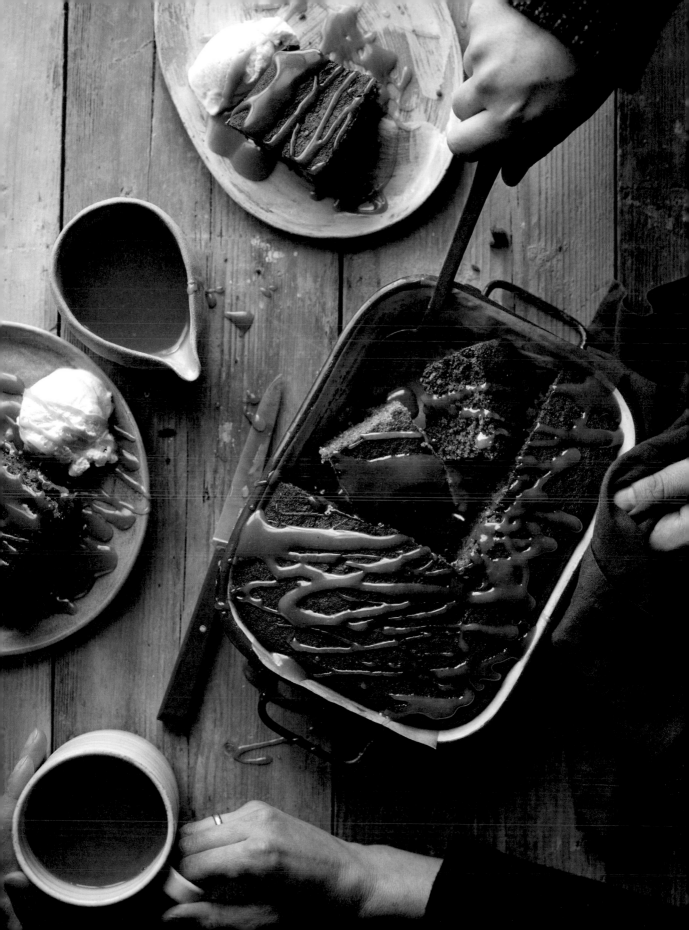

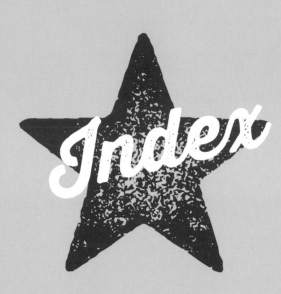

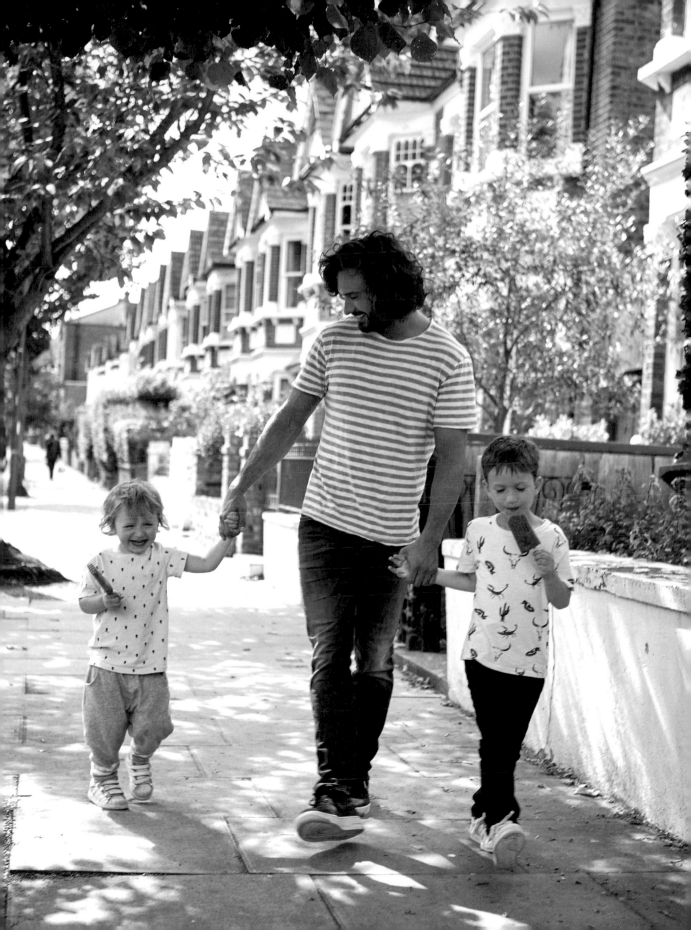

THANK YOUS

I want to start by saying a big thank you to all of my fans and followers on social media who made this book possible. Without your support I would never have got a book deal in the first place. When I stop and think about how many people are actually using my recipes it's hard to believe, but I'm so proud of it.

I also want to thank Bluebird and Carole, my publisher, for helping me create such an awesome book. It's been such a fun project making this.

I want to dedicate this book to my family and friends. The most important people in my life. The people who support me, believe in me and encourage me to achieve more. And big love to mentor and manager, Bev James.

Thanks Mum and Dad for always showing me love and support and telling me you are proud every day.

And to my brothers Nikki and George who are my heroes. And finally to the newest member of my family, the apple of my eye – Oscar Joseph Wicks.

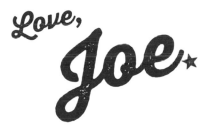

★ WANT TO SEE MORE RECIPES AND TRANSFORM YOUR BODY? CHECK OUT MY LIFE-CHANGING TRILOGY!

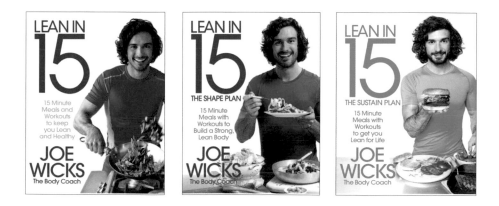

First published 2017 by Bluebird
an imprint of Pan Macmillan
20 New Wharf Road, London N1 9RR
Associated companies throughout the world
www.panmacmillan.com

ISBN 978-1-5098-2025-2

9 8 7 6 5

A CIP catalogue record for this book is available from the British Library.

Printed and bound in Italy.

Publisher **Carole Tonkinson**
Senior Editor **Martha Burley**
Junior Desk Editor **Natalie McCourt**
Editorial Assistant **Hockley Raven Spare**
Senior Production Controller **Ena Matagic**
Art Direction & Design **Jilly Topping**
Prop Styling **Lydia Brun**
Food Styling **Bianca Nice, Sunil Vijayakar, Lizzie Harris**

Visit **www.panmacmillan.com** to read more about all our books and to buy
them. You will also find features, author interviews and news of any author
events, and you can sign up for e-newsletters so that you're always first to
hear about our new releases.